How to Lose 100 Pounds

A realistic plan for losing weight

and changing your life!

P. Seymour

Contents

A Note from Paula…

Welcome to the compilation guide of my 6 book series "How to Lose 100 Pounds."

I don't know if you purchased "How to Lose 100 Pounds" because you do have 100+ pounds to lose or maybe less. Either way, I want you to know that this book series is a labor of love for me. I really hope that you can hear my heart throughout the pages as I strive to convey that I understand how you might be feeling. I know what it's like to feel like giving up. I know what it's like to let the weight control our lives.

PLEASE hear me when I say that you are not alone and you REALLY can change your life.

You are fully capable and you don't need a fad diet or a fast weight loss plan.

You do need to be able to believe in yourself and you need to know that YOU can create a very realistic plan that will have you losing weight AND enjoying your life as you do so. It is possible and it's not JUST about the scale.

I'm just a "regular" woman losing 100+ pounds who has found a number of strategies that work for me. In this book I'd like to help you develop your own little toolbox of ideas and resources that will help you to create YOUR plan for success, find the needed motivation, set some realistic goals, and develop your food and exercise plan. In the final section of the book, I also go over ways that you can get yourself back on track after a weight gain. I've been there myself and I know this can be a challenge.

Losing weight and getting healthy has affected every area of my life and I want that for you. I am not there yet myself, but I do know that SO much of the journey is about getting started and I can help you with that.

Let me walk with you as you create a plan for your own success.

These books are meant to be a series of blueprints to help you to find the motivation and tools that you will need to go the distance with any weight loss plan. I very much appreciate your reviews and comments as I love to put a name to those who are creating a healthy and happy life. I would love to be your biggest cheerleader if you'll let me.

To YOUR success,

Paula

Visit the site below to download my **FREE gift** to you - "Your Success Plan for Weight Loss." (And to be notified of new titles and special offers)

http://www.celebrateweightloss.com

Please also join us on FaceBook - there is a great, supportive group of people there:

http://www.facebook.com/howtolose100pounds

Book 1: Creating YOUR Plan for Weight Loss Success

A Note from Paula...

Have YOU had enough of being overweight?

Do you worry or think about...

— major weight related health issues such as high blood pressure, diabetes, heart problems?
— getting health insurance?
— fitting into an airplane seat or getting on to a crowded bus?
— a chair or bed collapsing under your weight when visiting your friends and family?
— being quietly judged and made to feel horrible about your size?
— kids and adults saying hurtful things about you?
— looking at the latest clothes & fashions wishing that you too could wear them and look good?
— feeling ugly & unattractive and thinking you'll never meet that special someone?

If you can relate to ANY OF THIS, then you and I have something in common my friend.

In Dec. of 2006 I weighed 278 lbs.
I was taking medication for high blood pressure.
I found myself getting winded going up one flight of stairs.
I was spending more and more time alone.
I was dealing with depression.
In general, I was feeling really bad about myself.

I finally hit rock bottom and knew that I had to make the decision to change my life and the direction I was headed.

I was SO sick of dieting and had FINALLY come to the conclusion that there really was NO magic fast formula for losing weight. I'm sorry if you've gone through that yourself but coming to that conclusion can really change things for you.

In Book 1, I want to give you some tools for creating that FINAL plan that can work for you AND allow you to do it with a smile on your face (well, most of the time!) and finally reach the place of health and happiness that YOU deserve.

This section is meant to be a blueprint to help you get up and running with your own weight loss plan quickly.

To YOUR success,

Paula

Creating YOUR Weight Loss Challenge

In December of 2006 I made the decision to change my life.

I was 37, single, overweight, unhealthy and very unhappy. I had made goals and promises to myself in the past, but I knew it was time to take a real honest look at where I was in my life. I literally began to have the thought that if I did not make a change, I might die.

A big fan of the TV show, "The Biggest Loser", I chose to create a challenge of sorts for myself. No excuses, as long as it would take....a plan to get fit, get happy, and create the kind of life that I felt destined to be living.

In this book, I want to encourage you to create your own personal weight loss challenge.

This is all about YOU, but I will make suggestions that worked for me and key areas that I feel will help to improve your level of success on this journey.

Key Areas and Suggestions for Planning YOUR Weight Loss Challenge:

1. The Big Reality Check

This does involve facing the scale, but we'll also talk about getting real and raw about the emotions of it all. How are you feeling physically, emotionally, socially? How has your life changed since putting on additional weight? This is not about blaming or making ourselves feel bad. We can only change what we are willing to face and acknowledge - this is the first step in the change that will be hugely positive in your life.

2. Do You Need to Schedule a Visit with Your Doctor?

This is part of getting real. I know for me where I was at physically scared me into making a change. I was at risk for many weight related issues and was already on blood pressure medication. Allow yourself to get real with the facts of the condition of your current health, knowing that it's only going to improve from this point on. I highly recommend before you start any exercise or drastic changes to your diet that you do consult with your doctor.

3. What is Your Vision for the "New You"?

How do you see yourself when you envision your healthy weight? Not only in how you will look but how you will feel. How do you go about your day differently? What people do you socialize with and what new kinds of activities do you see yourself doing?

4. Getting Clear About Your Motivation for Losing Weight

I think it's important to recognize the "why" behind the desire to lose weight and try to find some reasons other than the ones that are only physical. Sure it will be great to wear jeans again and feel cute when you go out, but how will this change your life day-to-day?

5. The Importance of Having Goals, Targets and Milestones

We're going to talk about the tools you might use to set your goals and track your progress. Having your ultimate goal and breaking it down into doable pieces will be hugely important in this process.

6. Preparation for Your Weight Loss Challenge

Here we'll talk about the actual tools that you may need as you get started. We'll come up with your fitness list and a suggestion for an initial grocery list as well as other tools that have helped me along the way.

7. Track and Be Prepared to Celebrate Your Achievements and Milestones Along the Way

Much of the importance of defining your clear goals has to do with being able to celebrate along the way as you achieve those goals and milestones. If you are like me, and have more than 100 lbs or so to lose, you can be assured that this is not going to happen overnight or in a few months. There will be year goal(s), quarter goals and monthly goals to work towards and you better believe that I'm going to encourage you to celebrate each of those along the way!

Are you ready? The time is now for you my friend. Don't wait until the New Year. You can have amazing achievements and a whole lot of momentum going as you ring in the New Year, knowing that this will be the year that you change the direction of your life.

I know you can do this! I can't wait to hear all about it.

The Big Reality Check

One of the first steps in planning your weight loss challenge is getting real with yourself. You cannot change that which you don't acknowledge and I know more than anyone how easy it is to be in denial when it comes to our weight and how we feel about ourselves.

I really want to encourage you to take the time to feel the full "weight" of what your excess weight has been costing you over the years. What things have you missed out on? In what ways have you stopped taking care of yourself? What is the dialog that happens in your head when you look in the mirror?

This is not about shame or blame.

Some Ideas for Getting Real

It's time to face the scale

Take a deep breath and get ready for the number. I promise you that the very hardest part of this process will be facing the scale and getting started. Once you know where you are at, then you can create a target. Once you have the target, it's forward march my friend!

If you are in a similar boat as I was in, with more than 100 hundred pounds to lose, the scale is probably not your friend. I very seldom weighed myself. In fact, at the time I began my weight loss challenge, I did not even own a scale. I believe this allowed and enabled my weight gain over the years. There is something about facing the number that causes reality to set in. Though this can be difficult, I believe that denial is never good and it will only allow you to continue to spiral in the direction you do not want to head.

So get prepared, muster up your courage and throw off your clothes. If you are determined to get the weight off, this is the hardest point right here. Once you have this starting number you will begin to enjoy stepping on the scale as you start to see the numbers go down. That's what you have to look forward to.

Taking measurements

While you're at it, get out that measuring tape. You will thank me later as the inches start to fall off and you look at what you've accomplished. Find key spots that you'd like to measure. I hit all of the these myself - upper arm, chest, waist, hips, thighs. Measure and record so that you know what your starting point will be. There will be times later when you might get frustrated with the scale. For me sometimes when the scale didn't move as much as I would like, I was happy to record an inch loss in key areas.

Journaling

I suggest that you use this time to do some journaling as well. At the very least, find a comfortable place to be quiet for a period of time and ask yourself the following questions:

1. What is your physical reality at this moment?

How much extra weight are you carrying? How difficult is it for you to do day-to-day things such as walking up a flight of stairs or tying your shoelaces? I know for me, I was faced with a general feeling of discomfort that affected my sleeping and how I felt about myself whenever I was around other people. I ALWAYS felt that I was "taking up too much space".

2. What health concerns are you facing?

Here I want to encourage you to take a look at your present situation. Are you facing diabetes or high blood pressure? Do you have a goal to get off of medications that you might be on? Let's take a good hard look at what scares you in this department. Before I began my weight loss, I can remember one day in particular when I honestly thought I was having a heart attack. It turned out to be an anxiety attack but it was the scariest thing physically I had faced and I actually remember thinking that I could die that day.

3. How is your social life?

Are you comfortable in social situations, or does your weight make you feel self-conscious? Are you constantly worried about what others might think of you? Does your weight keep you isolated? If single, do you feel that it hinders you from meeting that one special person or dating in general? If you do have someone in your life, has your weight affected your current relationship in any way?

4. How are you doing emotionally?

Do you have moments, days, or weeks of depression? What is the self-talk that goes on inside your head? When is the last time that you remember feeling good about yourself? What would it feel like to be confident again?

5. Finally, if this is something that is important to you (as a Christian it was to me), how do you feel that your weight affects your spiritual life?

I know for myself, I really want to be doing that which I believe God has created me to do. I know that includes being my best physically as it affects all other areas of my life. I don't want excess weight to be zapping energy that I should be applying to other bigger and more important goals for my life. Does any of this ring true for you?

I hope that this will get you started. Remember this is not about blame at all or beating yourself up. We are simply laying the foundation. I want you to be real so that you can build on the strength of that honesty to achieve the great things that are awaiting you!

Scheduling a Visit with Your Doctor

In the last section, we talked about facing the realities of what our excess weight has meant to our life. I know for many of us, the idea of going to the doctor can be the last thing you want to do, but I really want to encourage this especially if you haven't been for awhile.

This is part of getting real. I know for me where I was at physically scared me into making a change. I was at risk for many weight related issues and was already on blood pressure medication. Allow yourself to get real with the facts of the condition of your current health, knowing that it's only going to improve from this point on. I highly recommend before you start any exercise or drastic changes to your diet that you do consult with your doctor.

If you are feeling uneasy about facing the good doc, hold your head high and be ready to let him or her know that you are getting ready to make major changes in your physical health and you just want to be responsible and check in with them prior to your big roll-out! Seriously, they are there to help you, right?

Obviously, you know somewhat the health battles you are facing if you already have diabetes, high blood pressure or anything like this.

When I initially went to the doctor after not having been for awhile, here are the things that I was interested in...

1. An accurate weight check

I also suggest that you weigh yourself at home (if you already own your scale), right before you leave for the doctor and as you will there in the office. (without shoes for example) This is just to check the accuracy of your scale. Mine actually weighed about 2-3 lbs heavier than the doctor's did, but I never really did adjust for that as I was already into my weight loss at that point. So when I go now, it's always a nice surprise!

2. A discussion with the doctor about what a "healthy" weight for me would be

Throughout the whole journey, I've not really been attached to a specific number. I do follow the guidelines for what a healthy weight should be for my height. I figure that I will aim for mid to end of that range. I'm surprised though at how healthy/fit I actually felt at 160-ish, for example. By the "charts", I believe I would definitely be considered overweight if not still obese. By the way, my height is 5.5 so I don't have a lot of leeway in the height department.

3. A plan for getting off my high blood pressure medication

My doctor was great at listening to my desire to be off my blood pressure medication. We discussed my blood pressure targets and how I may be able to check this myself as I'm working through my weight loss. Many places such as Wal-Mart and various drug stores have the free machines where you can take your own blood pressure. I recommend that you do take it a second time after you've been sitting for a bit. I find that my first number is always higher but I think it is due to just running in the store. Actually I always make the doc take it a second time after I'm calmer as well. For me, I was able to cut down on the medicine in 2 stages. The first stage I could lower the dosage and eliminate one of the 2 medications I was taking.

4. A plan for my continued doctor visits

For me, I committed to checking in monthly to at least have my blood pressure monitored. Actually I began to look forward to these visits as my weight would be checked and there would be praise all around! I don't have insurance at the moment so if you don't for whatever reason, I can feel your pain there. Doctor visits can be expensive. I think a lot of places would be willing to work with you, so do check around if you are in this situation. I know that mine would allow me to pop in and get my blood pressure taken without charge.

Ten months and 75 lbs into my weight loss challenge, I got a clean bill of health from my doctor. WooHoo! I was completely off my medication by that time and he had been monitoring my blood pressure for a bit. This was a huge success for me and if you are battling health issues that are affected by your obesity, the changes you will see physically will be amazing for you as well.

Let's make our health our #1 priority as we move forward with your challenge!

Having a Vision for the "New You"

Here I'd like you to fast forward to the very best you that you can picture in your mind. Do NOT edit this image - this is where I want you to really dream about your future - the very future that you are going to set out to create.

Be careful not to get stuck on older images of yourself. For example, if you're around the corner from turning 40 (like I was!) I don't suggest that you put pictures of yourself from the high school prom on your fridge! Hey, we've come a long ways since the high school prom, right?!

You can envision a healthy, fit, slimmer version of yourself. For me, I really tried to replace older ideas for the desire to be thin with a vision of someone that was healthy, fit and strong. I knew that thinness would also be a part of that, BUT I didn't want to make that the end-all, be-all. If the goal is health and fitness, you can enjoy and realize this much earlier along in your journey. I began to feel strong and fit way before I truly liked what I was seeing in the mirror.

Here are some suggestions and I would encourage you to write these in your journal.

1. How will you look physically?

If you do have a fairly recent picture of yourself at a smaller and healthier size, you may want to get this out if you feel that it will help to inspire you. Picture yourself in a pair of jeans, a nice dress or whatever that article of clothing is that you've been dying to wear. Early on in my journey, a good friend really encouraged me to envision myself in a specific article of clothing. For me, I was picturing wearing a blue dress.

Fast forward months later, I was looking for something to wear for an outdoor summer wedding and I found myself in the dressing room looking at a reflection of me in the mirror that brought me to tears! It was the blue dress!!! Fitted at the waist, arms bare, the whole thing! Wow! Yes, create a vision for yourself! You will get there and I want you to have a moment like that.

2. How will you feel?

If you are in a similar place as to where I was when I started, you probably go to bed and wake up feeling sluggish. I was putting junk into my body that was totally depleting my energy level and I felt sick and tired a lot! Imagine feeling that you eat for energy and exercise because you enjoy the feeling it brings you and how much stronger you feel after. Picture yourself running up that flight of stairs while carrying your groceries.

3. How do you go about your day differently?

What things on a day-to-day basis will be different for you? Are there things, people and places that you currently avoid because of your weight or how you feel about yourself? What would you do if you had a bit more time in your day? I don't know how this works, but I can tell you that I thought I didn't have time to exercise on most days. What I found was that if I plan for some exercise during the day, I am SO much more productive and organized throughout the day that I actually get more done than the days when I don't exercise.

Picture these kinds of productive days for yourself. What would your perfect day look like? Let's move towards that.

4. How do you see your life changing socially?

Are there things that you do not get involved in currently because of your weight? Groups you'd like to join? Maybe you're single and you've been purposely keeping yourself out of the dating scene? Start dreaming and making the list of things you'd like to be involved with socially. You may surprise yourself and find a walking (or some type of exercise) group locally that you'd like to get hooked up with. I was very much a loner when I was overweight. I think a lot did have to do with how I was feeling about myself, but I have come to also realize that I do not have a real need to be very social. I am working on finding a balance with that.

5. Picture yourself 1-2 years from now if you do nothing to change your current situation with regards to your health and weight.

This is a hard one, I know. For me, I started when I was turning 37. In my mind, I looked ahead 3 years and thought about how I wanted to feel turning 40. I knew that if I didn't change or start to change something at that time, I quite possibly could find myself turning 40 being fat, sick, single and just all around feeling horrible. I knew without a doubt that I wanted something different...that I could create a different reality for myself. Don't dwell on this, but know that truly making the decision to change is half the battle. You can be in a completely different place one year from now.

Now that you have a clearer vision in your head for the "new you", get ready to put your pen to paper once more in our next sections as we delve a little deeper into getting really clear about what the motivations are for losing the weight and getting healthy.

What is the "why" behind the desire to lose the weight? This is what will keep you moving forward!

Getting Clear About Your Motivation for Losing Weight

In the last pages, we talked about how you envision your new healthy life. This is a picture of you physically as well as a vision of the way your day-to-day life could be different. Here, I want to get even clearer about this picture so that you are fully aware of what your motivations are for losing weight. I think it's important to recognize the "why" behind the desire to lose weight and try to find some reasons other than the ones that are only physical.

I will share with you some of the motivations that I personally came up with at the beginning of my weight loss challenge. Perhaps some of these will ring true for you as well? I hope that this will get you thinking about what is truly at the root of your desire to lose weight.

1. Physical

— I owned up to the fact that I had a difficult time walking even for 15 minutes. My body hurt, I was out of breath easily and my back hurt.

— I was living with a general feeling of discomfort every day.

— I was not sleeping well at night.

— I couldn't tie my shoes while sitting. (I needed to stand up and bend over to do it and it was hard)

— Public seats were often a tight fit. (restaurant, airplane, amusement rides - ugh!)

2. Health (actual and potential issues)

— I had high blood pressure and had been on medication for about 3 yrs.

— I had experienced some numbness in my legs, feet, and face at times - this was something that had really started to frighten me.

— I had experienced anxiety attacks and at one time had seriously thought that I was having a heart attack until I saw my doctor who diagnosed it. (BUT this was something that really brought home that I might be Lterally killing myself by not addressing my weight issue)

— I was dealing with some depression and I feel deep down that so much of it related to my weight and how I was feeling about myself.

— I knew that my obesity was putting me at risk for so many things. I feared diabetes and this is something that my doctor had really stressed with me as well.

3. Social

— Most often I didn't care about going out or being around other people. I had really begun to isolate myself.

— There were so many negative thoughts going on in my head during times with others. I felt embarrassed of my size and I often just felt that I was taking up too much space - ugh! How awful is that?!

— I was turning 37 as a single woman. Yes, I wanted to meet my future husband. I definitely felt that my weight was holding me back from this potential, because I felt that no one would be interested in me at the weight I was at...not just for the outward appearance, but what it said about my lack of discipline and concern for myself.

4. Emotional

— I had become such a good "faker". I knew how to pretend to be confident and happy when I was in social situations. People would not have called me shy and I didn't have a problem meeting people. I did like to be in relationship with others. However, this did not match how I was feeling on the inside.

— I was very uncomfortable in the heat. I didn't have the most appropriate clothes. I was too self conscious of my arms to wear sleeveless AND I couldn't wait to actually enjoy the — beautiful beaches in a swimsuit! I actually love swimming in the ocean and it had been ages since I've done that. (because I didn't want to get in my swimsuit in public)

— I liked to believe that I was OK with my singleness, but I had been crying myself to sleep some nights and if I was being honest with myself (and you) I'd been feeling scared of being lonely…scared that no one will ever love me or want to share their life with me. I knew that I really did want this and I wanted to bring my best to my future husband. This included the health and confidence that would come from losing the weight.

— It had been ages since I'd been able to shop in a "regular" store. I'm not saying anything negative about my usual Lane Bryant or Avenue for example, BUT I couldn't wait until I would be able to walk into The Gap or Old Navy and buy even their biggest pair of jeans! There are SO many more options available for people that are not overweight.

— My other biggest issue at the time had to do with finances and debt. I really believed that if I could tackle the weight issue and reach those goals, I could then apply the same motivation and focus towards my business and financial goals, eliminating the debt once and for all as well. I was thinking that there would be a lot of momentum that would carry over into every area of my life.

— I didn't know if my depression would be cured with the fitness plan and weight loss. I did believe in my case, that it was a large contributor of how I was feeling mentally and I was anxious to see how exercising and eating healthy foods would affect my mood. Forever the optimist, I believed that within a few months of beginning the weight loss challenge things would be much better in this area.

5. Spiritual (As a Christian, this was an area of my life that was an important factor as well)

— It drove me crazy that I felt that my life was not truly a testimony to the power of Christ in me.

— I wanted to bring my best to a relationship that I believed would exist in my future. This included my health, outward appearance and self esteem.

— I believed that my obesity was a result of a lack of discipline (among other things) and I knew that more discipline in my life could only help me to grow spiritually.

— I so believed that my weight issue was hindering me (that I was hindering me!) from being everything that God had intended for me to be.

I hope that my sharing my own motivations here will help you to get clear and honest about your own reality and the reasons you want to lose weight. I believe that taking some time to think about this (and writing it in your journal) will help you even more when it comes to being focused on your weight loss efforts. When times are tough and your discipline is lacking, you can get a boost by going back and looking at all the reasons that you want to lose the weight.

Goals, Targets and Milestones

We are starting to get down to the nitty-gritty of beginning the weight loss challenge. We've discussed the emotional aspects of why you might want to lose weight and I'm sure throughout this process you've been faced with some realities as to how the weight issue developed (or got away from you) in the first place.

Now it's time to start looking at our targets. What are our goals and the time frames that we can (realistically) achieve them?

When I began my weight loss challenge, I originally intended to lose 128 lbs that first year. This huge goal was largely inspired by the amount of weight that I saw people losing on the TV show, "The Biggest Loser". I wasn't being completely delusional in that I knew that they spent crazy amounts of time exercising, BUT I had a lot of flexibility with my schedule and the determination to do whatever it took to reach my goal. So, that was my intention when I started.

I revised this one year goal at the 6 month point (I'd lost 48 lbs by this time) to be 100 lbs and again at 9 months to be 85 lbs in the first year. I'm not saying that someone could not lose 128 lbs in a year. I know that people do lose these amounts of weight. I know for me, I began to really look at it as a journey and recognize that it was going to take some time. The important thing that I want you to realize here is that the target doesn't really matter as much as beginning the process.

You will gain momentum as you go and your targets may shift, but I promise that as you begin the process of getting healthy and losing weight, the length of time it takes to reach that ultimate number begins to matter less and less. Even though it has taken longer than I first anticipated, I am a completely different person at this point. I feel so much better about myself and the physical improvements to my life have been amazing. Mostly, I want to achieve that ultimate goal weight and size now so that I can finally start building a wardrobe that I know will remain with me.

So now let's spend a bit of time talking about goal setting...

1. Setting Your Ultimate Goal Weight

I suggest that rather than pull a random or old high school number out of thin air, that you visit and discuss with your doctor a healthy weight for someone your height, build and age. You can also find a number of healthy weight charts online.

2. Setting Your Time Frame(s)

Depending on the amount of weight you have to lose, this beginning time frame may be more or less than 1 year. If more than one year, I suggest that you decide on a realistic goal for year 1. This will be the starting point. If you start out wonderful out of the gate with your challenge, you will probably lose a lot of weight the first month or 2. I think it is attainable (if you have a lot of weight to lose) to expect that you could lose 10-15 lbs that first month or 2. I found that over time, I tended to average about 7-8 lbs a month in weight loss. Keep in mind that you should also have a goal to be gaining muscle which in the long run is ultimately what you want...strength and fat loss.

3. Tracking Method

Make this a pleasant experience for yourself. Go out and purchase that planner you've been thinking about, or pretty paper and colored pens. Don t just write these goals on scraps of paper. This is a process and getting organized will help! I used a regular 3 ring binder with dividers/tabs for each quarter. As techie as I am, I always seem to come back to good ol paper and pen.

4. Make This Goal Your Focus

If you have a lot of weight to lose, make this your #1 focus for a time. There is nothing more important than your health and I believe that getting healthy and fit will affect every other area of your life in a positive way.

5. Planning

Set aside time to set your goals. I set my monthly goals at the end of the month (quarterly where applicable) and my weekly goals on Sundays. In the morning, I create my list of goals for the day.

6. Celebrate Milestones

When you reach a goal, celebrate! The momentum you will feel will be tremendous and I promise that the first 5 lbs you lose will be the most important as the most difficult part (in my opinion) is getting started.

7. Plan for Revision

This has been one of the biggest learning points for me and something that I hope I can carry into every area of my life. I do tend to be somewhat of a perfectionist and I think this has definitely been a detriment to past weight loss attempts. I would start doing some kind of program, fall off the wagon and ditch the whole effort.

This time around I really recognized the power of forward motion. The day-to-day choices I make do not have to get me off track if they are not a choice within my plan. So one night of pizza and chicken wings no longer turns into eating out 4 nights that week. 5 lbs gained over a weekend away does not need to signify an upward trend of weight gain upon my return back home. It's very important to break your goals down and look at them from month to month and quarter to quarter. If you need to revise your year goal, go ahead....remember that you are moving forward and that is what really matters!

I hope that these tips will help and inspire you to start creating your plan...your challenge for the new you and the New Year! Hey, you don't have to wait for the New Year to get started!

Preparing for Your Weight Loss Challenge

The countdown has begun. It's time to get yourself physically prepared for your weight loss challenge. Please don't let the purchase of items stand in your way of getting started. Begin with what you have now. You can always add to your plan later.

This is a list of some basic items that you may need. These are things I personally use (or have used) on a day-to-day basis.

Some Motivational Resource Suggestions:

— Anthony Robbins' ULTIMATE EDGE™! (general motivation to change your life) (In association with Guthy-Renker LLC's ANTHONY ROBBINS' ULTIMATE EDGE™!)
— general motivational books
— books based on The Biggest Loser TV Show

Progress Related:

— a scale that measure in 0.1 lb increments
— measuring tape to record your decrease in inches

Exercise Related:

— comfortable walking shoes (I love ASICS shoes)
— floor mat (if you will be doing any floor work)
— set of dumbbells (5 lbs to start, working up to 10 lbs)
— iPod (not essential, but I love listening to something while walking)
— 8 Minute Ab workout DVD (I do this 5 days/wk and I think it has made a HUGE difference to my waist/core!)
— Pilates DVD (I do this 3 days/wk and again feel that it has had a great impact - I use Ana Caban Beginning Mat Workout by Living Arts)
— comfortable walking clothes (sweats, shorts)

Food Related:

— scale for weighing food
— measuring cups, spoons
— notebook for food diary (to count calories)
— low calorie cookbook(s)
— calorie counting book (I use The Biggest Loser Calorie Counter)

Grocery List: (this was my initial grocery list - feel free to modify this and make it your own)

— lots of vegetables: lettuce, carrots, cucumber, broccoli, green beans, potatoes
— lots of fruit: apples (I love Fuji), bananas, strawberries, blueberries, oranges, kiwi, pears
— skim milk
— margarine
— low calorie (wheat) bread
— cereal (Shredded Wheat, Oatmeal)
— eggs
— lunch meat (turkey or ham)
— cheese (slices, shredded low fat Mexican, parmesan, string cheese)
— pasta and pasta sauce
— rice (I like Basmati)
— tortillas
— taco seasoning pack
— beef (ground sirloin for lowest fat/calories)
— chicken
— other meat/protein options
— low sodium canned soup

If you think it may be difficult to figure out what you will be eating, I would start out your challenge by actually writing down your meal plan for a week. I realize that this may require more planning depending on your situation. As a single person, the food was pretty easy for me to sort out day by day. If you are also cooking for others, this may be a bit more challenging. I suspect the whole family will be eating healthier as a result of your challenge. Please keep in mind that I am not really advocating any special diet here. We're simply going to go back to the basics with balanced meals from the food groups.

Happy shopping!

Tracking and Celebrating!

One of the biggest reasons that I suggest you have a written plan for your weight loss challenge is so that you can very easily identify your targets and celebrate your milestones along the way.

Certainly achieving your ultimate weight loss goal will be a HUGE accomplishment, BUT there is no reason why you cannot and shouldn't also celebrate the smaller goals met along the way. This will help to keep you disciplined and the discouragement will be lessened if you have a lot of weight to lose. If you are like me, and have more than 100 lbs or so to lose, you can be assured that this is not going to happen overnight or in a few months. There will be year goals, quarter goals and monthly goals to work towards and you better believe that I'm going to encourage you to celebrate each of those along the way! Let's learn to enjoy the process of getting healthy and fit!

Begin with your ultimate weight loss goal. Think about the amount of weight you will have lost when you achieve this goal. The more you have to lose, the more cause for celebration, right? For me, the idea of losing 145 lbs (or so) before my 40th birthday brings me to a vision of doing something fantastic to celebrate. I'm still dreaming of what this might be, but I'm quite sure it will involve some sort of travel and quite possibly some sort of physical challenge. One idea, for example, is a bike trip through Italy. WooHoo! How cool would that be?!

Think about ways that you may like to celebrate. Another idea may be a fantastic and well thought out shopping trip. Finally the sizes will be stable and you may even like to treat yourself to a personal shopper or stylist at this point.

So, you should start to dream a bit about what this celebration will look like for you. Reaching your weight loss goal is not a small thing and putting your health first should be viewed as a major accomplishment.

So, what other milestones might we celebrate?

For me, a few of my weight loss milestones included (in this order):

1. Losing my first 10 lbs (week 4)
2. Losing 20 lbs (month 2)
3. Being under 200 lbs (month 11)
4. Losing 100 lbs! (1 yr, 4 months)

Some other milestones included:

1. Adding cycling to my exercise routine (month 7)
2. Getting off my blood pressure medication (month 10)
3. 1000 miles logged on my bike (month 10)
4. Being able to shop in "regular" size stores
5. Buying and wearing a pair of jeans
6. Various biking mileage records (to date 45 miles!)
7. Feeling awesome at my 20th High School Reunion (1 yr, 8 months)

Tracking Your Weight Loss

I suggest that you weigh yourself at approximately the same time every day and with the same amount of clothing on for accuracy. For me, it's first thing in the AM before I eat anything and in the nude. (hey, I'll take every bit I can)

Once you have your starting weight, you can put your plan into motion. If you have a lot to lose, I think it is very realistic (assuming you are determined and diligent in your efforts) to expect to lose anywhere from 8-12 lbs that first month. This is where you really start to get some momentum going. If you can imagine getting that first 10 lbs off, this is totally doable for 30 days from now. 10 lbs can make a big difference in your life emotionally. You need to start getting some traction and the first 10 lbs can get you hooked!

Some people say that you should really weigh in once a week or so...that every day is not a good thing. Personally I do weigh myself every morning and for me, it's a good way to follow patterns of weight loss and to see how eating certain foods affects my weight from day-to-day. For example, I can have a great low calories day, but if there is a food that is higher in sodium, such as canned soup or ham, that might show on the scale as weight gain for a day or 2. BUT since I weigh myself every day I can see that numbers go back after my consistency within a few days.

Mind you, there have been days, weeks, months ;) where I've wanted to throw the darn scale out the window!! That's when you really have to dig deep, change up your routine and look at your inches, your clothing and how you are feeling. This will happen as well and I will talk more about how to deal with a weight loss plateau in a later book.

Now, on to the celebration portion...

What are some "rewards" or things you can do to celebrate your achievements along the way? Certainly there will need to be new clothes as you eliminate your larger sizes. One thing I realized along the way was how infrequently I had been doing nice things for myself. As I neared my 100 lb mark, I decided to celebrate this milestone with a new hair style (cut and color) and professional make-up application. (and the purchase of new make-up) This was a reward that celebrated my achievements as well as helped with my perception of the "new me" that I was becoming.

I know many people say that you should not reward yourself with food and I do agree with this in general. However, most months after I do my monthly weigh-in (assuming it's been a good month with the weight loss) I do treat myself to something. Most often this is pizza and chicken wings. Be very careful here though as it really depends on if this will cause a spiral of food challenges for you or if you can handle the one night treat. With good planning, I have found that this can be done. If your weight loss journey will be a long one, I think it's almost necessary to plan for some treats as totally eliminating everything you ever loved from your diet can backfire on you.

This part of the planning stage is fun! Please enjoy it and think about how great you will feel at each stage of your journey.

Book 2: How to Find the Motivation to Lose Weight and Get Healthy

A Note from Paula…

I think it's quite possibly easier for someone who is 100 lbs overweight to find the motivation for losing weight than someone who has much less weight to lose.

When you are 100 lbs overweight a lot of things really suck! Let's just be real for a moment and recognize that obesity colors nearly every aspect of our lives. At least this is how it was for me. I don't want to mislead anyone into thinking that getting fit will make all of your problems go away. Of course that is not true at all and I'm also not suggesting that someone who is obese can not also be happy with different aspects of their life.

While I was in denial about feelings, health and creating a better life for myself, I became a very good dreamer.

If you have a lot of weight to lose, I bet you can relate to this.

In my dreams of being healthy, fit and good looking, everything was better. I could imagine having a relationship, traveling and feeling different when I walked into a room at a party. I could imagine the miracle of having that better life.

When I finally made the decision to lose weight and reach for that lifestyle, I knew that these dreams had to become the driving force behind every daily decision that I made as it related to my health and weight loss efforts.

In order to follow through on the plan you developed in "Creating YOUR Plan for Weight Loss Success", you are going to need to get extremely motivated and this motivation will come from different places for different people.

Only you know what thoughts, dreams, images and other resources will truly help you to dig deep in order to realize the success you deserve.

In Book 2, I'd like to help you develop your own little toolbox of motivational ideas that will help you to have the drive to climb that mountain of weight loss and see it through for yourself.

This section is meant to be a blueprint to help you find the motivation that you WILL need to go the distance with any weight loss plan.

To YOUR success,

Paula

Without Motivation You Will Fail

Let's get real for a moment. If you are like me, you've probably tried to lose weight many times. Quite likely you can start off with a bang and then before you know it as soon as the urge/craving/thought comes to you, you're off and running for the ice cream or whatever strikes your fancy in the moment.

This has been my experience and I can tell you that you need a plan for digging deep when those moments strike.

I can also tell you that it probably won't always work - sometimes, you'll cave to the urge. BUT a slip up doesn't have to set you back if you have a plan. We'll cover that in a later book.

For now though, I want to talk about your plan for getting through those moments. Where will the motivation come from to REALLY stay the course?

We can start off with our lists knowing our big reasons why we MUST lose the weight once and for all…only to be derailed with a single decision.

You need to have a strategy in place for when you're in the moment and faced with a yes or no choice.

For me, this mostly seems to occur in the evenings while watching TV. So knowing this is one thing for sure. How can you choose to NOT throw your hands up and give in to the late night snack when all of the sudden - in the moment - you simply don't care.

I love to have something visual and many of the suggestions I have for you will be visual ones. You need to literally have a picture - real, or one you can easily conjure up in your mind - that WILL be your motivation to make the right decision in the moment.

Know Your Story, Then CHANGE It

Every life comes with a story...and a possibility for a great adventure. ~ Kobi Yamada

I've been a fan of the TV show, "The Biggest Loser" ever since it began. I once heard popular trainer Jillian Michaels say the following to one of the contestants as she was struggling on one of the pieces of gym equipment.

"This is a story in your head. None of it is real. All you have to do is change your mind."

What?! Wait a minute! This was the biggest female contestant that they'd had on the show to date. If she felt that her body couldn't do something, was that incorrect? I mean we do have physical limitations...don't we?

Hmmmmm......

Shortly after this, I was doing the Jillian Michaels: No More Trouble Zones workout as I'd been doing for weeks. Every time I would do this dvd, there were certain exercises that I couldn't (really?) do all the way through. One of those was the dreaded surrender move where you hold your dumbbells over your head while kneeling and raising to standing position.

So, on this particular day I realized that maybe this "I can't" business was only a "story in my head"....maybe if Jillian was right about the contestant and she had been completing amazing fitness tasks - maybe I could do this silly surrender move all the way through!

OK, go figure! Changed my story, completed the move!

53

Could it really be THAT easy?

Change the story in your head, CHANGE YOUR LIFE, even?

I remember the day I decided to buy a bicycle. I had lost about 48 lbs at this stage of my weight loss journey and was weighing in at about 230 lbs. I had been thinking about this for awhile, but I honestly had the idea that it was something that I needed to wait for. After all, fat people can't ride bikes, can they?

I made the decision to go to the bike shop and literally stood there talking to the salesman with hands on hips saying…"OK, Am I too fat to ride a bike?" Of course, he denied this and sold me a bike that completely revolutionized my exercise routine! When that story in my head changed, the weight started coming off even more rapidly because I found a type of exercise that I completely enjoyed! Riding the bike that first time has become one of my favorite memories during this journey to health, fitness and freedom.

My weight loss journey DID begin with a decision. There was a story playing in my head at that time that had all the makings of a very sad ending…a sad life. I had tried so many times to lose weight and the story I was telling myself was that I could only fail again, but was that real? Could it be only a thought and could I decide something else?

What is the story you are telling yourself today? Have you failed time and time again at losing weight? Are the words you hear in your head, reality? Or are they simply words?

If other people have lost the same weight or more than you have to lose, is it possible that you could also achieve success?

Can you change YOUR story?

I know YOU can! Decide today that YOU deserve every positive thing that you could imagine coming your way...regardless of the past, regardless of the story, regardless of the obstacles that are before you.

What's the NEW story in your head...begin to live THAT story.

Your WHY

I will always encourage you to be positive and to think and speak in ways that will uplift and empower you to achieve your weight loss goals. If you're like me, you've had enough self loathing and negative talk to last a lifetime. Let's be done with that now.

Health

For a moment though, I think it is important to look at all of the negative aspects of your obesity. What are the extra pounds costing you in your own life. For most people, the easiest thing to look at first - well, at least in terms of the most obvious thing - is one's health. If you are already dealing with health issues related to your obesity than you are well aware of what it has already cost you and what the ramifications could be to NOT losing the weight.

Your Family

Are you a parent? If so, your weight and health probably does affect how you interact with your children. We all know that kids have a lot of energy. Keeping up with them can be difficult even for the most fit of parents. You probably also feel the pressure of the kind of example that you are setting for them when it comes to healthy habits.

Your Work

Does your weight or health affect your career? Are you truly able to perform at your highest capacity? Even if your job does not involve activity, chances are that your weight does affect your self esteem which could alter your overall performance at work.

Your Relationship/Romantic Life

Are you single? This may be the most obvious of social issues for someone who is overweight and single. No matter how people might speak to the contrary, it can be difficult to understand why someone would be attracted to us at our current weight. This is as much an emotional issue as a physical one.

Relationships With Friends

Have any of your relationships suffered due to your weight and how you feel about yourself? Sometimes our friends can also be "partners in crime" if they are also dealing with weight issues. If this is the case, it's important to be around people who will support you and who won't sabotage your efforts. Getting fit together can be a great thing if you both understand the need for support from one another.

Social Life

How is your social life in general? When friends invite you out on the town do you say no because you've got nothing to wear? Do you decline parties because you imagine people looking at you and thinking about how much weight you've put on? As you get fit and start to feel better about yourself, you'll probably also be more inclined to take part in social activities.

What dreams are you giving up?

What will your life be like in 5 years if nothing changes or you continue to gain weight and be unhealthy?

What will your life be like in 1 year, if you start to make positive changes now that will bring you closer to your dreams?

What is YOUR why? What are you determined to see for your own life in 1-2 years?

Having Vision

Now let's take that "why" factor to a whole other level. This part is fun!

What would you do if your weight, health and fitness were not an issue? Dream BIG!

These dreams may be the things that really motivate you for moving forward and do not discount anything. This will change as you start realizing success and you might discover goals and dreams that you wouldn't dare to imagine.

For example, you could be that person that goes from barely getting off the couch to competing in an Iron Man or race of your choice. This is just an example of something that could happen once you connect with that potential athlete living inside of you.

Not everyone has dreams of being an athlete and that's OK.

My big example has been my dream to travel and create a location independent lifestyle for myself. I always wanted this but being 100+ lbs overweight left me feeling like I would never even really enjoy it until I lost the weight. My dream for this type of adventure did not include feeling self conscious and unhealthy.

What are your dreams? Regardless if they have anything at all to do with your current weight or health, I can almost guarantee that reaching your health and weight loss goals will carry with it a sense of self confidence in all areas of your life. Do you want to feel unstoppable? That WILL be you!

Your big WHY and your vision for what you want in your life will be that driving force and motivation that will help you to dig deep to realize your weight loss and health goals.

Document Your Starting Point

This step might be a difficult one for you.

We all know that most people who are 100 lbs (or maybe even 20 lbs) overweight do not enjoy having their picture taken. I would also cringe when I saw photos of myself. Dare I say I never liked any of them.

This is the step that you can do now and then completely forget about it until either you need it or you are celebrating your wild success. Please trust me that you will thank me for this later.

Muster all of your courage and your best friend or a loved one to capture your "before pic". As much as we're used to trying to hide our fat with dark colors, baggy clothes and certainly never the willingness to be captured on film in our bathing suit, this is the time to be really true to yourself. If you can muster the courage, take several pictures that show your current weight. Consider taking pictures from different views - side shot, from behind and also one in your bathing suit. I suggest you take several because in the event that you do decide to show these to people later (AFTER your success!), you will probably want several to choose from.

Keep 1 set of "big" clothes as you lose weight. This can make for the most amazing success picture and when you later put these clothes on, it can be extremely motivating as you see just how far you've come in your journey.

Here are some additional things that you might want to consider doing that can help with your motivation throughout your weight loss process.

Take a video of yourself. Take a video of you talking to yourself. In the video, describe how you are feeling at this moment and how you never want to go back to this place again. If you can, really connect to your feelings at this current weight.

Write a letter to yourself that also really connects to your feelings. Tell yourself all of the ways that you've hurt yourself in the past and the hopes and commitments you have for the future. Write about the reasons you are committing to a healthier lifestyle and the vision you have for a changed life and dreams realized in the near future.

All of these ideas can be tools that you can pull out later if you find your motivation diminishing. When you look at that picture or watch yourself in the video, it can be that one thing that will help you to get back on track in your weight loss efforts.

Choose the things that will work for you, but don't dismiss this step.

Starting a Fire

Losing a lot of weight is like starting a fire when it comes to momentum and how you feel along the way.

It can take some work to get a good fire going. You know that it only takes a flame and a bit of effort at the beginning before you have a nice warm blaze going. One might begin with a small piece of paper which then catches the smaller kindling on fire. Once those few pieces of kindling wood start to burn, it's only a matter of time before those few big logs turn into a nice steady blaze and from here, short of putting the fire out, you can plan to watch it burn for hours.

I think this is similar to how it is when getting started with a big weight loss goal.

I'd say the hardest part IS getting started. Getting started requires the simple but pivotal decision to change your life…to light the fire and put the plan in motion with commitment and the dedication to do what it takes to make your life look different in the near future.

The weekly goals you make and the daily decisions you choose are like the kindling in the fire. To being with, just get them moving…each decision and action you take towards that positive outcome will help to build your momentum. These may seem like the smallest of decisions to begin with, but making commitments that you know you can follow through with at the beginning can mean so much for your confidence and the acknowledgment that you have what it takes to keep promises to yourself.

Here's what I mean as an example…If you are starting where I was with more than 100+ lbs to lose, you've probably not been doing too much in terms of healthy choices, let alone physical activity.

Here's the way to set fire to some of those smaller things that will lead to your larger goal of doing cardio 5 times a week. (as an example)

Your week 1 commitment might be to write down the negative things you are saying to yourself and create positive affirmations that you can start to say. As another action step, let's add a goal to take a daily vitamin. (as an example)

Week 2 might be to keep a daily log of what you are eating and to be more conscious of the choices you make. Perhaps you can add a goal of drinking 8 glasses of water each day.

These are things that will not be too "painful" in terms of change, but they will get you in a mode of being more conscious about your daily habits.

Week 3 might be the time you start the buildup to some regular exercise. If you've not exercised at all and it's difficult for you, maybe your goal is to walk for 15 minutes 5 times throughout the week. Make it achievable to start and know that just getting started might be challenge enough for you right now. Let yourself complete the goal and feel a sense of achievement as you move on to your next stage of the plan.

These small things are going to build on one another until you have a full fledged fire burning. This is a metaphor for your goals but a similar thing could be said for your metabolism as you start doing more exercise and eating foods that nourish your body.

You can start off your plan having done nothing for ages but eat poorly, sit on the couch and tell yourself horrible things, to looking back over the month with the following accomplishments - taking a daily vitamin, drinking 8 glasses of water a day, exercising for 30 minutes 5 times a week and eating a big salad 5 times a week. This is just an example, but you can see where I am going with this.

How do you think you are going to feel after a month like that? I predict you would be going into month 2 with a blazing fire.

Month 2 can have you rolling up your sleeves ready to make exercise goals and create menus that will give you energy and get you inspired.

Everything you want to achieve can really begin with a series of small goals and commitments like the examples here. Think about the smallest of changes that you could begin with and get started ASAP with those.

Finding Support

Many people have a difficult time losing weight and feeling motivated when they are completely alone in their efforts. If you feel that this could be an issue for you, be proactive in your desire to find some support. There are many places where you can find like-minded people who will be going through the same things that you will be facing. Here are some ideas for getting support either locally or within an online community.

Local Support Ideas

MeetUp

MeetUp is a great online community board where you can find all kinds of local interest groups. Once you sign up and enter your location information, you can begin searching the groups within your immediate area and according to your interests. You'll find groups on all different types of topics and you can even organize your own group if you don't find one to suit your needs. Of course, there is a greater selection if you live in a bigger city, but many locations do have groups. Think about finding a group organized around an activity such as walking, biking or hiking. You might also look for a women's group or mommy group as another example.

meetup.com

Various Weight Loss Programs

Many people turn to a paid program that has local support in order to lose weight. I am not advocating any one weight loss program and in my own recent efforts, I did not choose to invest in a specific program but I will mention a few in case that is the direction you decide to go.

Weight Watchers - This is a very popular program and one that I have personally tried in the past with some success while involved in the process. They do incorporate real food which is nice and the program is very realistic and doable. There is also a big support element to this which includes weekly weigh-ins and meetings with other people. You can even join this program online these days and participate in the online support groups.

weightwatchers.com

Jenny Craig - This is another popular program that provides regular support with a consultant. With Jenny Craig, you do also purchase their food so this is one thing to consider in your overall strategy. Many people may prefer to start out with this because there is less work involved when it comes to cooking and knowing what you can eat each day.

jennycraig.com

Nutrisystem - This is another option that includes pre-packaged food. This also includes a lot of support via an online member site.

nutrisystem.com

Your Doctor

Of course one of the first things you'll want to do before starting any serious weight loss plan or effort, will be to schedule a visit with your regular doctor. Most likely your doctor will be one of the first people to get on board with your efforts to get healthy and lose weight. If you have some serious health concerns or goals that you are targeting, utilize your doctor and their office to be able to monitor your progress when it comes to such things as your blood pressure for example. Your doctor should also be able to recommend a good nutritionist if this is something that interests you as you begin your journey.

Mommy Group

If you are a parent with small children, search locally for some type of mommy group that you can engage with. Many time moms with young children love to get out with the strollers and walk together when the weather gets nice so this could be a great way to get some exercise and support.

Church

If you belong to a church or other spiritual organization, seek support here as well. There might be a small group that meets to exercise or support one another when it comes to health and weight loss. Sometimes seeking prayer and counsel in this area can help greatly with your efforts if spirituality is a big part of your life.

An Accountability Partner

Enlist the accountability and support of a friend or relative. This can be very helpful especially if the other person is also working towards the same goals. Having that understanding and support for one another can really help to get you through the rough times when resolve weakens.

Online Support Ideas:

Twitter

Twitter can be a great place to find a community of like-minded people about any topic of interest including health. This is free and easy to use. Sign up for an account and using various search functions you can start finding other people that are tweeting about health and weight loss. Once you begin following a few people in this area of interest, look at who they are following and who is following them to find other people to start following yourself. Jump in and join the conversation and soon you'll find a great little online support network.

twitter.com

Blogs

Via Twitter and regular online searching, find a great group of health and weight loss related blogs to begin following. If you have a Google account, you can use the Google Reader to subscribe to a blog's RSS feed. This is great for organizing and staying up-to-date with the ones you'd like to follow. You can also participate with many blogs by posting comments about the blogger's articles. Many times a blogger will also have a Twitter and Facebook account so it's another way you can begin to be part of a larger community.

Facebook

Facebook is a great way to find people to connect with who are also trying to lose weight and get healthy. When you visit a blog that you enjoy, look for a Facebook button to "like". Once you visit the Facebook page you can also follow other people and other pages that are related.

facebook.com

Pinterest

Pinterest is one of the newer online communities that is growing at a rapid pace. Like many of the other online boards, you can find people here to follow by searching various topic ideas. Later we'll discuss another cool idea for how Pinterest can play a part in your weight loss motivation.

pinterest.com

YouTube

Like the other social networking sites listed above, you can use the search function of YouTube to find and subscribe to people who are also on a journey to get fit and lose weight. This site can be especially fun because the power of video helps to really feel that you can connect with a person and share in their struggles and celebrations.

youtube.com

Various Weight Loss Communities

The above is not an exhaustive list of the various online resources that can help you in the area of support with your weight loss goals. A simple Google search for weight loss sites and forums can turn up many different options that may work for you.

Reading for Motivation

If you are someone who enjoys reading, arm yourself with plenty of good books and other reading material to help motivate and inspire you throughout this journey.

You're already aware of Kindle books and the instant gratification that now comes from being able to order an electronic book to read within minutes. Research the areas of health, fitness and weight loss to find other popular books that people are purchasing and commenting on. Amazon is a great place to do this type of research because you can read reviews and glimpse the inside of the book before you make your purchase.

You may also want to look for general books on motivation and goal setting. Two authors in this arena that I really appreciate would be Anthony Robbins and Brian Tracy. Once you develop a list of authors that you like, you can also find many related books.

There are also online book recommendation resources that are fun to follow and participate in. Check out Goodreads as one great example.

goodreads.com

Blogs

As mentioned earlier, set up your Google Reader application to organize the RSS feeds for the various weight loss and health related blogs that will inspire you throughout your journey. It can be very motivating to read the stories, struggles and celebrations of other people who are going through the exact same situations as you.

Quotes

Start a collection of favorite quotes that inspire and motivate you. Pin them up on your wall, in your workspace and on the refrigerator to help to keep you motivated to reach your goals.

Set a goal of reading one new great book a month (or a time period that is reasonable to you) and choose something that will keep you inspired and moving towards action when it comes to achieving your goals.

Listening for Motivation

If you are not a big reader, this section of ideas may appeal more to you. Even if you are an avid reader, adding some audio resources to your motivational toolbox can only add to your success. There are so many great places where you can find good audio books and Internet radio these days.

Audio Books

If reading is not your thing, you can find many of the main authors books in an audio format these days. One of the biggest sites for this would be Audible. Here you can start a subscription and download books every month to listen to while driving or on your iPod while exercising for example. You can sample most of the books here before you purchase.

audible.com

ITunes and Amazon would be other big sites where you can buy individual audio books.

apple.com/itunes/
amazon.com

Podcasts

Listening to podcasts on my iPhone has become my favorite thing to do when I am walking for exercise. Choose something that will help to inspire you to be fit and healthy or to reach another one of your big goals that has to do with the vision for your future. As an example, since such a big part of my vision includes travel and location independence, I listen to podcasts from other people that are already involved in this lifestyle. This helps to keep me motivated to work towards my goals. You can find podcasts on a wide variety of topics within the iTunes Store.

apple.com/itunes/

Motivational Courses

Some of the main authors that I mentioned before, such as Anthony Robbins and Brian Tracy, also have motivational courses that you can purchase that are in an audio format. If this is something that helps you to be successful, it can be well worth the investment to add this to your list of motivational tools.

Music Mixes

Many people get inspired by upbeat music, especially when they are working out. Create your own music mixes that will help to get your energy up and your heart rate going. Check out 8Tracks or similar websites to find out what other people are listening to when they create music mixes.

8tracks.com

Meditational Tracks

If you are someone who is spiritual, you certainly might consider a time of prayer or meditation to be an essential part of your journey. Check out 8Tracks for ideas on mixes that people have created to help with meditation or quiet times of prayer. Additionally, you might consider finding podcasts that have to do with sermons or spiritual topics.

Affirmations and Prayer

There is a lot to be said for the words we say to ourselves in our own head. As an experiment be very conscious as you go about your day to be aware of how you are speaking to yourself. Are you calling yourself names that have to do with your being overweight such as fat and lazy? Are you speaking to yourself in ways that you would never speak to another person? This can be very eye opening to say the least.

Once you catch yourself in this bad habit you can start to change it. For some people, the best way may be to actually write out some positive affirmations to speak aloud throughout the day. If you can write down some negative things you say to yourself, you can start by creating positive statements out of these.

For example, if you find yourself saying something like:

"I have so much weight to lose that it's going to take forever for me to get there"

Change it to:

"Every day I am creating more health in my life and the weight is coming off in a way that is healthy and best for my body. It will take as long as it takes and in the meantime, I'm going to enjoy the journey."

Create your own list of positive affirmations that you can say to yourself throughout the day. It can be a good idea to start and end your day by speaking these affirmations out load. It may seem a bit silly at first, but if you're willing to give it a try you might start to see a change in how you feel about yourself and speak to yourself internally.

Prayer and Meditation

If, like me, you are a Christian or you practice some type of spiritual beliefs, you may want to consider bringing prayer or meditation into your daily routine.

This can be an incredible part of your journey and can help you to find strength from within when the going gets tough. Centering yourself daily on the things that are really important can be critical to your success and happiness.

You can find specific bible studies or various spiritual books that specifically have to do with health or weight loss. If spirituality is an important part of your personal life, that can be a beneficial thing to commit to as you begin your own goal of getting fit.

Create Something Visual

For many people, creating a visual representation of your goals can have a very powerful effect. This can be as simple as pinning up photos and favorite motivational quotes to creating very cool online vision boards that you're able to share with others in a like-minded community if that is something that would be useful to you.

Images of Yourself or Others That Inspire You

Do you have pictures of yourself at a lower weight that would inspire if posted where you could see them? Be sure that the picture matches a goal that is attainable. For example, if like me you're struggling with weight at age 40, I wouldn't advise putting a picture up of a fit you at your high school prom.

Maybe you are inspired by others who have the type of body you'd love to work towards. I would encourage you to put pictures up that will inspire you to carry on towards your goal. If you want a strong and lean body like fitness star, Jillian Michaels, put her picture where you can see it when you work out.

Vision Board

A physical vision board can have whatever pictures inspire you to reach your goals. Aside from putting pictures and quotes that will inspire you to reach your fitness goals, you may also want to include items that inspire you towards the dreams and visions that you outlined earlier.

For example, if your ultimate dream is to get fit and healthy so that you can buy a backpack and take off on a trip around the world, your vision board might include images of the various destinations that you want to visit on your trip.

If your goal is to own your own home with a gourmet kitchen to cook from, your vision board might include images that represent your dream home and kitchen.

Your vision goal is fully about representing you and all of the awesome things that you are working towards. Place the images where they will benefit you the most. Maybe its in the same place where you work out or maybe its in the kitchen to help when faced with making food decisions.

Computer Wallpapers

If you spend a lot of time on your computer, another great motivational tool is to choose a nice inspiring wallpaper or set of wallpaper to watch on your computer screen. You could also consider putting together a little slideshow of your own images that show fitness and health.

Favorite Quotes

Many people find great inspiration by reading quotes on a daily basis. If you find a quote that really speaks to you, consider showcasing it in a way that it inspiring to look at. I would recommend that you find and dedicate one quote to be a mantra of sorts as you begin this process of changing your life.

I will share with you the favorite quote that I have right now pasted on a binder that goes with my goals of being fit and location independent.

Our deepest fear is not that we are inadequate.
Our deepest fear is that we are powerful beyond measure.
We ask ourselves,
"Who am I to be brilliant, gorgeous, talented, and fabulous?"
Actually, who are you not to be?
We were born to make manifest the glory of God that is within us.
And as we let our own light shine,
We unconsciously give other people permission to do that same.

~ Marianne Williamson

Feel free to borrow this quote for yourself as I believe it speaks so well to many of us that are living less than the life we deserve.

Graphs or Checklists of Your Goals

In my quest to get fit, I've realized that I am like a kid when it comes to having a visual chart to star, sticker or check off.

My sister and I once did a biking challenge together - 500 miles on the bike over the course of a few months. I didn't really get on board until we plastered our individual (decorated) graphs on the fridge to track where we both were. Then it became game on! We loved coloring in our squares after coming in from that 20 mile bike ride.

This is something that might work well for you also. Consider making a good old fashioned chart for specific exercise goals or other goals that you want to achieve on a daily basis.

Pinterest

Pinterest is one of the most exciting new social media platforms to hit the online communities. We talked about it earlier in terms of using it for a source of community and support. Here, I'd like to talk about it as a way to create online vision boards for the things that will inspire you throughout your journey.

You can basically take the above ideas and translate them to different boards online within your Pinterest account.

Sign up for an account and spend some time looking at what other people are doing to get some ideas. You can create multiple boards for things that inspire you or you might have one basic board to serve for your weight loss inspiration.

Some examples might be a board that has different outfits (and accessories) pinned on it to inspire that fashionista in you. You can start designing your new wardrobe before you even lose your first 5 pounds. Talk about inspiration and fun!

You could also find websites with images that inspire you and collect these images all in one place on your own board.

If like me, you are dreaming of travel, create a board with images of your favorite travel destinations.

Back to the home/gourmet kitchen example, begin a board with pictures of your favorite kitchen appliances.

Here is the link to Pinterest where you can check it out and starting pinning your way to motivation.

pinterest.com

I hope this gives you some good ideas of ways that you can use visual images and quotes to keep you inspired on your journey to lose weight. When it comes to motivation, it's important that you build up your own tool chest of items to keep you motivated along the way, especially if your journey won't be a fast one.

Documenting Your Own Journey

You may want to consider documenting your own journey as you work to reach your heath and fitness goals. It has become much easier to do this online these days and depending on your level of comfort with technology, it can be as simple as you need it to be.

Keeping a public record of sorts can be beneficial to you as well as other people. If you have a desire to help other people with their own weight loss challenges, this is an excellent reason to start a blog or some form of online community. People will value your experience and also it can have the added benefit of increasing your own accountability when it comes to achieving your goals and keeping your motivation up.

This book is not a blogging or online business course, so I will not go into great detail with this. I will, however, provide some ideas and links below where you can get started and find more information on how to do so.

Start a Blog

Blogging has become very big nowadays and it's very easy to get started. If you are looking for minimal technical skills needed, you can set up a free blog on Blogger, Tumblr or an account on Squidoo. There is a lot of information available at the various sites and by doing a little research so you should be able to get up and running pretty quickly.

blogger.com
tumblr.com
squidoo.com

Another big platform that many people use is Wordpress. Wordpress is also free and doesn't have to be very technical if you just want to get a basic blog going. If you do think you would like to grow your blog into a bigger platform over time, I would highly suggest using Wordpress and hosting your own blog. You can find out all about Wordpress here and there is also a lot of training available on this topic.

wordpress.org

Start a Facebook Fan Page

With the huge increase in the popularity of Facebook, you can not go wrong to get started here. Creating a Facebook Page and community is a great thing to do along with your blog or even on its own if you'd like to start with this. Note that I am referring to a page here in contrast to a regular personal profile. You do need a Facebook profile first, but then once you have that you can create pages through the profile, but not connected to your own personal contact/friends in any way. Here is a link for more information about Facebook pages.

facebook.com/pages/

Build a Community on Twitter

As spoken about earlier, Twitter is a great place to start connecting with people and also build your own community. If you think it will take awhile to get your website or blog up and running, you can start with Twitter first. By the time you have your blog ready to go, you can already have a nice list of followers to check out your articles and information when you post your links.

twitter.com

YouTube

We also mentioned YouTube earlier and this is another great example of a way you can start sharing your own journey with other people. Technology has gotten so doable lately that you can shoot good quality videos with your small camera or smartphone. If you like the idea of using this type of media outlet, video is an excellent way to connect with other people because videos can be so personal in nature.

youtube.com

There are other social media and blogging platforms that you could use to start documenting your weight loss journey, but this list is some of the more popular options.

Personally I recommend that you document your journey because it really can help others and you may want to take things to the next level even by writing your own book one day in the future.

Treat Yourself Now

I'm not sure if I am alone in this way of thinking but I have a feeling that there are others that can relate to this idea.

When I was extremely obese, I was not only NOT taking care of myself physically regarding food and exercise, but in so many other ways as well.

Looking back, I didn't really feel that I deserved anything good or pretty in my life. I was always waiting until I lost the weight to treat myself to anything (other than food). This includes the obvious such as new clothes and new hair styles. I also really didn't treat myself with even the things that didn't really have to do with my body. For example, I'd rarely paint my nails, let alone book a mani/pedi appointment.

Looking back, I realize how silly and actually detrimental this was to me.

I remember going through a stage of epiphany. Actually I was seeing a therapist at the time that helped me to recognize some of this. By the way, I am a big advocate of therapy and come from a place of believing that anyone can benefit from seeing a therapist at one point or another in their life. If, like me, you've spent a great deal of your life with a lot of excess weight, there are probably emotional issues to deal with in one way or another. We all have our "stuff" so I'm not suggesting there has to be an overall trauma that would trigger someone to gain all of the weight.

How are you treating yourself these days? Aside from the obvious which may include what you are eating and how much or how little you are exercising, what are you doing that treats yourself in a positive way?

Not to sound trite, but do you truly love yourself right now, right where you are…love handles and all?

I know you've probably heard it before, but reiterating how important it is to love and value yourself regardless of your current weight or fitness level can give you a big jumpstart in this process you have ahead of you.

It can be difficult to get started, but the first step is becoming aware of the way you talk to yourself and changing some of that language.

For many of us dealing with obesity, we truly deny where we are at emotionally and physically. I would do almost anything to avoid looking in a full length mirror and then be shocked when I just happened to catch a glance in a shop window on a particular day. Its likely this would have sent me into a tailspin of depression for a time…and if I'm being honest, could most likely lead me to a round of fast food stops or a pint of Ben N Jerry's.

I remember when I started experimenting with being more in touch with myself and my body physically. I tried to treat myself with little things like getting my nails done or buying a new body lotion. I had another Aha moment when I realized just how much putting on lotion connected me to the body I had grown to hate. This was a good thing and I really started to speak to the good things I was doing for myself when I would go through the process of putting on lotion for example. I know it might sound small, but if you're not doing it, it can make a big difference.

Treat yourself now - in all ways. I'm not suggesting you even spend money. Start with your words and the way you talk to yourself. Instead of worrying about how others see you, remind yourself of all the good things you are doing for yourself and how committed you are to your process for getting healthy.

I can remember a moment being in the checkout line at the grocery store when I had lost some weight but was still considered overweight for sure. My cart was filled with nothing but healthy and nutritious food. I was getting ready to hop back on my bike because I had made this grocery trip part of my exercise routine for the week. Instead of worrying about people judging me for what was in my cart or how I looked, I remember just feeling pride in the fact that I was now making healthy choices every day. Not 100% perfect days, by any means, but a series of good choices that would lead to ultimate success.

Start treating yourself well today and find reasons to pat yourself on the back. Use your daily successes to motivate you to keeping reaching towards the awesome future that you deserve.

Book 3: Goal Setting for Weight Loss

A Note from Paula...

Here is the part in the series where I admit to being a bit of a geek when it comes to planning, goal setting and systems. I actually love this stuff. I love to read about it. I love to try different strategies. I love it when the power of goal setting results in REAL success.

Whether you're trying to lose 100+ pounds like I am, or any amount of weight, having clearly defined goals can make the difference between moving forward to success or throwing in the towel.

I vote for giving yourself the very best shot at success by first having a very clear target that you will then work towards.

Goal setting and planning is not difficult. If you have any interest at all, you've probably read a few books on this topic before now.

I'm all for reaching for goals that are BIG - we all need those types of goals. However, what I speak about in the upcoming sections on breaking down your goals, might surprise you. I'm all for losing big numbers on the scale week after week. It is possible for sure. We watch it on TV and we read about it in books that promise solutions/diets that result in losing x number of lbs in 7 days.

Having said all that, and knowing that I want you to be healthy and fit as fast as is possible, I'm going to be asking you to make a shift of sorts in the way you're thinking about your weight loss. I can almost guarantee you that if you will allow yourself to change your thinking about this, you will almost instantly feel a sense of relief and a real conception that you can finally do this for yourself once and for all.

I can say this because I've been where you're at...looking ahead at a goal of losing over 100+ pounds and desperately wanting to believe that I could do it, yet feeling that the journey would just be too long and too hard.

I'm not going to say that it will always be easy, but I predict it will NOT be as hard as you might think. I also predict that you will feel 100% better than you do right now before you even lose a fraction of what your ultimate weight loss goal is. You will feel 100% better 2 weeks from now…you will feel better for JUST having started because you will have a target and a plan moving forward that is now going in one direction.

In Bock 3 I'd like to help you to develop your own strategy for setting the goals that will help to propel you to reach success with your own weight loss.

This section is meant to be a blueprint to help you to develop a strategy for goal setting and create a plan that is actionable and doable for you.

To YOUR success,

Paula

Effective Goal Setting

For a goal to be effective, it should be concise and easy to measure. If you have any experience with goal setting, you are probably aware of this concept.

I like to further think about the things that I have the most control over. To illustrate this idea, I do have a goal weight in mind, but prefer to think of the actual numbers as targets. This is because it is more within your control to reach the individual goals, such as the amount of calories consumed and weekly exercise sessions, rather than to hit the actual number. Sometimes there are weeks that the scale just doesn't move and I'd rather you patting yourself on the back for crossing off all of the healthy choices on your weekly list than beating yourself up because a particular number is not yet showing on the scale.

The numbers and inches will come, its just that I want you to focus on the measurable things that are going to help you get there over time.

In terms of weight loss goals, there will be different things within your strategy that you will be able to target and measure. Of course you will have a target weight or range for your ultimate weight loss goal. You may have other goals, such as getting to a certain dress size or fitting into a particular pair of favorite jeans. Those all become great little gifts and rewards that you will notice along the way for sure.

The more measurable goals that you can set and achieve on a weekly and daily basis are the ones that I'd like you to focus on, especially when you are getting started.

Planning Your Strategy

I would suggest that you make the process of setting your goals and planning out your strategy an enjoyable one.

Decide how you want to map out your big plan, your goals and track your progress as you move forward. For some people, this might mean buying a new journal, downloading one of the apps mentioned later in the book, or starting a folder with documents on your computer. It doesn't really matter what method you use and keep in mind that this can also be a work in progress as you find the things that will best work for you.

When I started, I created a Word document with a list of my bigger targets. This included my ultimate weight loss goal and then as I further broke it down into what would become my year 1 goal and my 1st quarter goals.

I then set up different documents for my monthly goals and those get assigned to weekly/daily goals within my weekly planning system.

Set it up so that you can easily pull up your list of goals when you need that shot of motivation or direction.

Your Ultimate Weight Loss Goal

There are two things that you need to do before you commit that goal weight to paper.

1. Gain absolute clarity as to where you are currently. Yes, this does mean facing the scale.

2. Do the research and preferably visit your doctor to determine a realistic and healthy weight range for your height, age and build.

It's time to face the scale.

Muster up your courage, throw off your clothes, take a deep breath and step on the scale. This may just be the scariest part of this whole process, but you can't start mapping out your strategy for success unless you know exactly what your starting point is and exactly where you are headed.

While you're at, I suggest that you take your measurements also. Determine the measurements for the key areas that you want to track and then it will be up to you how often you might want to check-in with that or if you even do it at all until you reach your goal weight. What you measure is up to you, but I'd suggest thighs, hips, waist, chest and upper arms.

There will be times along the way when you do everything right during the course of weeks regarding your calorie and exercise goals, yet that scale refuses to move. Trust me when I say there has been more than one occasion when I've wanted to throw that blasted thing out the window! Sometimes when you hit a plateau of sorts on the scale, you will find your body has an inch loss. I noticed a pattern myself over time with this.

Know where you're headed.

I would always recommend that you schedule a visit with your doctor before you change anything to do with your typical routine. This is particularly important if you are dealing with any health related challenges as you'll want your doctor to advise you when it comes to your own strategy for losing weight.

If you're anything like me, you're probably somewhat resistant to going to the doctor. I think there is a fear of the disapproval and the knowledge that they are going to want to talk to us about our obesity and the importance for getting the weight off.

This may be another "take a deep breath" and suck it up event. It really is important that you know exactly where you stand currently in terms of any potential or known health issues. Go in to this visit with the determination to bring your doctor aboard as one of the integral team members regarding your weight loss plan. Let him or her know that you want to get the weight off in a way that will be the healthiest for you. Listen to your doctor's advice and ask that they give you a healthy weight range that you should be working towards.

Most likely, you will want to pick your goal weight in the middle of that or on the lesser end of it. I suggest you start at the top of that range. There will be plenty of time as you get nearer that weight range to determine what really feels the healthiest for you.

At this point, you now have your actual weight and measurements. You've chosen your initial goal weight and determined the magic number that is your ultimate weight loss goal.

I guess for some of us, this may also be pause for a deep breath. Congratulations on taking that first step and getting out of denial!

Now let's move on to how you're going to break that ultimate goal down in a way that will only lead you to victory!

Breaking It Down

Earlier I talked about preparing yourself to make a mental shift of sorts. Here's where that comes in.

Let's start thinking now in terms of a time frame.

First of all, if you are someone who has 50 lbs or less to lose, congratulations! Yes, you heard me right. You can totally conquer that and you can do it within the year...probably sooner.

If, like me you're looking at 100+ pounds, I know you want that off yesterday...all of it. You're probably thinking that you're going to fully commit to a diet and exercise plan AGAIN and get this weight off as soon as possible. It's probably hard to imagine that you could even be on a diet for more than a year.

Here's where the shift comes in and please really feel the importance and reality of this.

Where were you at with your weight one year ago? What about 2 or 3 years ago? For many of us, life probably wasn't all that different. We may have been depressed, constantly trying to start a new diet, vowing to do things differently, hating out bodies and ourselves...you see where I'm going with this? What if this time you made a decision that wasn't about how fast you could get the pounds off, but was all about getting healthy and fit and moving towards a goal that was 100% realistic?

What if you knew that a series of the smallest choices over the next year would result in a complete change for your life, your health and how you feel about yourself?

I'm going to say again that I am a BIG believer in setting and achieving BIG goals, reaching for the stars and achieving the impossible. I DO believe all those things for you.

I just know that after beating ourselves up, sometimes for years, the very best thing we can do for ourselves is to create a series of goals that will lead to success. This means choosing goals that may seem small at first, but will lead to much bigger things than you could even think about right now.

This might also mean that if you have 100 pounds to lose, you cut yourself a small break this time by saying - what do I know that I absolutely can lose each month? We all know that people can and do lose lots of weight really fast. You've probably been able to do this yourself. What if instead of setting a goal of 10 pounds a month, to start out with you determined that your first target would be 5 pounds a month. Could you do that pretty easily? I'm guessing that by cutting back on the eating out and adding exercise, most people could easily lose that 1b and a bit each week without hardly thinking about.

So, what if you had a goal to lose 5 pounds a month? 1 year from now, that means you could be 60 pounds lighter than you are today? Do you think that would make a difference to your health and life in general? You better believe it would!

So I'm saying even IF you have 100 pounds to lose, it doesn't have to be the struggle its been in the past. You don't have to be fanatic and change every single thing in your life all at one time to create real change. Heck if you have a goal to lose 5 pounds a month, you can even have dessert or plan to go out to eat one meal a week I'd say. You will quickly see what will work for you in terms of reaching your weekly and monthly goals but it definitely doesn't have to be as drastic as you might think.

The real key is to make your plan manageable and create small goals that will lead to long-term steps towards your healthy lifestyle, as opposed to a diet you go on and off.

Your One Year Goal

Based on what we were talking about in the last section, if you have 50 pounds or less to lose, I suggest you set it as a one year goal or less if that makes sense and is realistic to you.

One thing to realize with your goal setting is that even though I am suggesting that you do get great clarity and put the pen to paper when it comes to committing to your goals, you don't need to worry about anything being set in stone.

I know that if you have 100 pounds to lose and your one year goal becomes a 60 pound loss, chances are you will be doing a revision to that goal because you really will lose the weight much faster than 5 pounds per month.

As you start to set and achieve all those smaller goals, you're most likely going to thrive on that feeling of accomplishment and really want to push yourself to up the ante a bit.

For our one year example goal, let's say that you want to lose 60 pounds. One year from now you will be 60 pounds (or more) lighter than what you are today. Really let that sink in and you might want to revisit (or look at) Volume 2 where we talked about the importance of staying motivated and how you can keep that picture of being 6o pounds lighter constantly in your head or visually in front of you in some format.

You can do this! Let yourself imagine how it will feel to lose that amount of weight.

Once you've set your one year goal, put it on your paper, in your planner, on your computer or however you'd like to record your goals and accomplishments.

For your one year goal, you now have your target. I would also suggest that you set one or two other one year goals that might go along with your new healthy lifestyle. Is there a race you can imagine doing? Some type of walk-a-thon or hiking trip with the girls? Maybe you'd like to learn a new sport such as tennis or golf. This goal doesn't have to be something that you immediately start on physically, but it can be a picture to keep in front of you of something you are working towards.

You might also choose to set a goal that you can imagine doing when you are feeling better about yourself emotionally or perhaps in social situations. Maybe you have a goal to be more active in the community or to participate in some type of local organization. Really try to push yourself a bit with these goals.

Next we're going to break your one year goal down into your first quarter goal.

Quarter Goals

Typically I create my one year goals for the start of the new year, BUT you will be starting now and that's OK. Imagine how you will feel going into the new year with the knowledge that losing weight actually doesn't have to be your complete and only resolution.

If you were beginning at the first of the year, you'd have your one year goal and then your four quarters would begin in January, April, July and October. If you're close to beginning a new quarter, I say give yourself a bit of time (not more than a few weeks) to prepare and get ready to jump in. If it's not that close, just jump into the current quarter and we'll call that your pre-quarterly goals.

So with your quarter goals, we're just going to break down whatever that one year (or less) goal is.

Using 60 pounds as our example for a one year goal (or target number), our quarter target could be 15 pounds. You could also take a look at where you are starting from and be more or less aggressive with that number.

The reality is, if you have a significant amount of weight to lose and you are highly motivated to begin with, chances are you'll lose that 5 pounds in a week or two! If this is the case, you won't just take a rest of course…you'll dig in and then celebrate at the end of your first quarter when you realize how much sooner you are going to be able to lose that 60 pounds.

This weight loss target should be recorded for your quarter goal. I like to call the actual number a target as opposed to a goal because the reality is that the number is more or less not under your control and I really want you to focus on your actions to hit those target numbers as your true goals.

I would also suggest that you take a look at your other one year goals to determine how you might best get started with those during your first quarter. Typically if your goal involves some type of activity or event, these first goals might include a research phase. If the other goals are physical in nature, it may also include the very beginning of your new fitness routine with an aim to be much more active going into your second quarter.

Other ideas for quarter goals and what has worked for me, would be to think of some good goals involving the food that you will be enjoying and the new exercise that you want to add to your current routine.

This could include things like cutting back when it comes to eating out or you may want to experiment with adding new foods to your current diet. Depending on how picky of an eater you might be, another goal might be experimenting with new vegetables, proteins or recipes in general. If you live in certain areas that offer cooking classes, a great quarter goal could include finding a class to enroll in and this might also incorporate a social goal for you as well.

I'll let you in a little secret here which I find to be quite silly now. Growing up, I pretty much hated all cooked vegetables. I carried this belief right into my adulthood and pretty much didn't even think about an alternative to not liking cooked veggies. I did enjoy several raw vegetables so would get some nutrition once in awhile from salads.

When I began to plan out my food and calorie goals I determined that I was going to look for some recipes and tips on cooking vegetables properly and then try a wide variety over the course of the first few months. Needless to say that once I learned I could cook them in a way that did NOT result in complete mush (go figure, right - like anyone would like that!), I really found myself enjoying a wide variety of vegetables that I now eat on a regular basis. So trying new foods might be a perfect quarter goal for you too.

For most people, (and after a discussion with your doctor of course) I would think you should definitely be planning to head into your 2nd quarter goals with a pretty active fitness schedule on your weekly calendar. I am not here to tell you what that should look like, but I definitely want to encourage you to start being more active than you are now. I will be covering exercise tips in another book, but here I'll just say that you should really try to tap into something you do enjoy or something you might be able to learn to love.

For me that exercise turned out to be biking, but I also really enjoy walking which can be the perfect exercise for most people who are just getting started.

So, think about where you want to be at in terms of your fitness goals going into your second quarter. You may not really have a good idea of what you'll be able to do, but just remember there is always room for revision, so begin with something that is realistic and also something you can reach for.

An example of this for someone who has 100 pounds or more to lose and hasn't been exercising, might be the following.

At the end of my first quarter (will assume you have a full 3 months here), I will be walking a minimum of 30 minutes a day, 4 times a week. Then over the course of the next few months, you're going to back into that goal and probably hit it way faster than month 3.

Now that you've set your quarter goals, you're ready to take the next step in breaking it down further.

Monthly Goals

You've set your one year goals and further broken that down to your first quarter target weight and goals.

Now is when the real fun begins. Keep in mind that when you are looking at a month, we're potentially talking about significant change in a relatively short amount of time.

In our example of a 60 pound one year target, this first monthly target will be 5 pounds. Now, let's just be real here for a minute. I want to only set you up for success which is why I'm suggesting that 5 pound target. I don't really know where your head is at with this whole weight loss plan yet. I know after I had created my plan and began to utilize some of the motivational suggestions I shared with you in Volume 2, I was highly motivated to lose that first 10 pounds.

Here's the truth. If you have a lot of weight to lose, no one else is really going to notice a 10 pound weight loss, BUT you will notice. I can almost guarantee you that when you hit that first real benchmark, there is no stopping you because it will feel so amazing. And here's the other truth…if you are highly motivated like I was, you'll probably make some changes to your diet, start exercising and that 10 pounds will definitely be off within the month. I think my first month I lost somewhere between 12-15 lbs.

I also want to point out here that I am NOT talking about some crazy diet or feeling hungry or deprived all the time. I know that you can do that for awhile and you can lose weight by doing that, but trust me when I say to reach your longer term goals you have to be able to create a livable every day solution that feels healthy and good to you. This, my friend, includes the odd treat and what I like to call an "organized pig-out".

Not to get off course here because I will definitely be covering my strategies for handling cravings and planning "treat days" in the later volume about food suggestions, but I just want you to keep remembering that this is about smaller changes over time. It is not about going from eating fast food twice a day (yes, there was a time in my life when I did this), to suddenly existing on salads, water and grilled fish every night. Not that there is anything wrong with those particular food choices. They will have their place, but your diet and food choices can and should be as varied as you want to make them.

Also, you will want to look at your additional quarterly goals that do not have to do with your monthly weight loss target.

If you have a quarterly goal to locate the race or event that you want to sign up for by the end of the year, this first month may be all about doing your research online to see what you might be interested in and to locate sites where you can get further information. This first month could also be a research time for locating a cooking class if that were one of your longer term goals, for example.

For our example quarter exercise goal of walking a minimum of 30 minutes a day, 4 times a week by the end of the quarter, a good first month goal might be to be walking 15 minutes a day for a minimum of 3 days a week. I know that doesn't sound like much but for someone who is very overweight and not used to any exercise, that goal can change your life. Trust me when I say that getting outside and doing any amount of movement is going to help you so much. Not only physically – and it could be uncomfortable, by the way - but helping you to get into a different state emotionally as well.

I will talk about a quick example here that also shows how determined I was when I started at 278 lbs AND how determined I know that YOU can be.

Create a 30 Day Challenge

I often like to do these 30 day challenges with myself. It may or may not involve my health or fitness. Sometimes these challenges are business or productivity related. When I started my commitment to this plan to get the weight off and change my life, I decided to do a challenge of walking 60 minutes/day for 30 days straight. Yes, I was kinda crazy and doing exactly what I'm suggesting you don't do. I knew I "could" do it and I also was betting on the projected payoff of what I believed would be incredible momentum.

I started off on Day 1, iPod in hand ready to conquer a nice 60 minute walk. For some reason, I didn't actually realize that it had been ages since I walked for 60 minutes at one time, not to mention the amount of weight I had added to my poor body. So feeling sweaty, tired and horrible I realized that this was to be a lesson to me about revising and making something work for me with my health and goals in mind. I decided that I could pretty comfortably walk around the outside perimeter of my apartment complex in about 15 minutes. The new plan was born! I would go on to complete my 30 day challenge and much of the 60 minutes walking each day was done in 4 blocks of 15 minutes.

Do you think I felt good about myself and had an amazing sense of accomplishment at the end of that month? You better believe I did!

Maybe you could attempt a 30 day challenge yourself. It can be something entirely different from an exercise challenge. As an example, you could do a 30 day challenge around drinking x number of glasses of water each day. Or maybe the challenge would be about eating a vegetable of some sort each day. You get the idea. Have fun with it!

The monthly targets and goals will then be further broken down into your weekly goals.

Weekly Goals

Sitting down to do my weekly goals has become an enjoyable part of my routine. See, I told you I was a bit geeky like that. These days, this includes pulling up my favorite app on the iPhone which is the 2do app for managing my weekly and daily items. (I link to that later in the book for you.) I do my weekly goals on Sundays which seems logical to me, but you should do whatever works for you in terms of your weekly tracking.

This is really where the rubber meets the road so to speak. Your determination to accomplish the goals you set for yourself for the week will largely determine your ability to follow through with them each day and ultimately achieve the results you are wanting.

I will encourage you to make certain that your goals for your first week are completely doable. Don't get me wrong...I'm picturing you in a similar position that I was in when I started. This might mean little to no exercise happening and a diet consisting of two different fast food runs each day. If this is anything that you can relate to, your week one goals should be things like the following suggestions:

— a commitment to writing down everything you eat during the course of the week (this will serve a purpose in helping you to be less in denial about your current intake)

— taking a daily vitamin

— drinking 4 8 ounce glasses of water each day (working your way up to 8 of these)

— eating 2 big salads during the week

— going for one walk during the week - minimum of 15 minutes

These are just ideas and you certainly do not have to choose a certain number. Choose things that you can feel great about completing and things that are moving you towards a more healthy life.

All of these small building blocks and goals will matter. You are taking steps. You are on a journey and you will get there if you persevere and stay aware.

Especially when you are first doing this, I urge you to NOT overdo it. I do not want you to feel any ounce of negativity at the end of your first week. This time is ALL about setting yourself up to accomplish something and begin to feel the momentum you are going to need to see this through.

Don't get me wrong…as you go about your week feeling better each day, you may surprise yourself and WANT to go for a walk or check out your apartment gym. Do this and count it as bonus! It is also all about your pushing yourself just a bit so you will have a clearer understanding about where you are at and the things you can add for week 2, week 3 and so on.

PLEASE keep your promises to yourself! Honor your commitment to these weekly goals and do what you need to do to MAKE them happen.

I say this especially to the woman (or man) who is 100+ pounds overweight because I KNOW that you do not often do this. It is a gift for you to give yourself. Start honoring yourself and creating the life that you DO deserve.

I want that for you and I want you to want that for yourself.

Daily Goals

This is where many of us mess up.

I used to mess up with my daily goals ALL the time prior to REALLY making the decision to change my life. I maybe would have gone through the motions of setting my monthly and weekly goals which would include exercise and eating goals. The day would start out fine and before I knew it, I'd find myself on the couch watching TV suddenly not caring at all about my commitment and obsessed about a new idea in my head to give-in to a craving. It was literally as if a switch had been pressed.

Is this something you can relate to?

I think in the moment, the thought comes into our head that one bowl of ice cream (pint of ice cream!), a few cookies (box of cookies!) or an extra sandwich (or 2!) is NOT really going to matter in the grand scheme of things. We're already SO overweight that it will hardly be noticed. It is SO easy to just give in to our old and comfortable habits. For many of us, these habits of eating certain foods during certain times really do make us feel comfortable.

How badly do you want to change right now? How important is it for you? This is why I wrote the previous book on motivation. I KNOW that you are going to need something in front of you to pull you through times and days like this…when you forget WHY you really want to lose the weight, get healthy and change your life.

I began to play a little game inside my head…sometimes on a daily basis. Somehow you have to be able to pull yourself out of those times when you go a bit blank when it comes to your goals. YOU need to create that for yourself. You will need to create some strategies for overcoming these urges.

Don't get me wrong here. I am not perfect and I do cave at times, but being self aware is really so much of the battle won. Our real danger is going into denial about it. THAT is how someone like me managed to gain 100+ pounds.

Here are some suggested strategies for achieving your daily goals and promises to yourself:

— Begin your day with a clear list (not huge) of what your goals are. I prefer to do my list in the morning, but you may like to prepare yours the night before.

— As much as you can, try to get the most important items crossed off early in the day. For me this includes exercise. I do so much better when I complete this in the morning as opposed to later in the day. Of course, you will have to structure your own days according to what will work for you.

— Know what your daily menu will be. Planning is critical when it comes to organizing a good eating plan. It's a good idea on a weekly basis to be sure that you have the groceries and ingredients for the foods that you want to prepare during the week. This is especially critical when you are just getting started because you will be less likely to give in to cravings if you are not wondering what you should be eating.

— Know your weak moments and plan how you will handle them. For me, I'm at my weakest during the evening while watching TV. I'm pretty convinced that it is just a habit but it can be a strong compulsion nonetheless. I have done a few things to help me during this time. I've done a 30 day challenge where I have an eating cut off time during the night. It can be hard but typically I can keep the commitment and remind myself that if I am really hungry, I can have an early breakfast. Most often, I just plan a snack for the evening. Usually this is something sweet like a chocolate Fiber One bar or a Root Beer float with low calorie ice cream. (I'll be providing more food examples in a later book about the food portion of your weight loss plan).

— Recognize "true" hunger and if it's real don't deny yourself. Make a good healthy choice that will satisfy your hunger. I do not believe that you need to be starving yourself or feel hungry throughout this process. You should be striving to feel satisfied and energized by the foods that you are eating. Sometimes from one day (week) to the next you may truly require more calories. This can be due to an increase in exercise or for many women it can be a result of your menstrual cycle. Keep aware and make good choices and you should be fine adding a few calories to your day when you need it.

— If you make a mistake (and you probably will...I know I do!) keeping your promises for a certain day, the MOST important thing after you make that decision will be what you do the next day. Do NOT wait until Monday to "get back on track". Do THAT the very next day. Remember you will achieve your long term weight loss goal by honoring your daily commitments. Every day is the chance to move one step closer to that ultimate goal you have for yourself. Do not let any single day defeat your week or any single week defeat your monthly goals and you will achieve success.

Build Revision Into Your Plan

I would say that I can be quite the perfectionist at times and I promised myself while creating my weight loss plan that I was going to do something different this time. If you've tried and failed to lose weight in the past, recognize that you need to be open to new ideas and giving yourself a little grace sometimes.

You've created your ultimate weight loss goal/target. (based on a healthy weight range)

You've then created quarterly goals, monthly goals and you are all set to knock off the daily items to achieve those weekly benchmarks.

The truth is, life will happen. Things will come up that will throw you. Be ready for the challenge and do your best to constantly be in a state of forward motion. Sometimes forward motion towards your ultimate weight loss goal can simply mean not going the other direction. For example, if you are planning a week vacation you're probably feeling a bit nervous about how it will fit into your commitment to lose weight because you may have gained weight on previous vacations.

How can you plan for success and have an awesome time away? I think this is the perfect example of practicing your new healthy habits with the goal of not gaining (or not gaining more than x lbs) while you are out of your "normal" routine. It can definitely be a time to splurge on meals you wouldn't normally eat or a few drinks that you normally wouldn't have, but what can you carry with you? Can you plan some activity while away? Maybe its simply a daily walk to enjoy your environment. Can you create a plan for eating that includes a 80/20 rule? I'd bet that if 80% of your food choices are good and healthy, the 20% splurge will not cause a weight gain that wouldn't quickly be reversed once you are back into your routine.

The key really is being able to plan and to not be rigid when life calls for flexibility.

I also think you need to have times throughout your plan where you will sit down and modify your goals when it is necessary. This could be because it is taking longer to hit your targets, but it could also be a modification because you are losing your weight much more rapidly than what you had originally imagined. THAT kind of revision is fun!

For example, let's say that your ultimate weight loss goal is to lose 100 pounds and you've set a one year target weight loss of 60 pounds. You've further broken that down into a quarter 1 goal of 15 pounds with a monthly target of 5 pounds. If you absolutely smash that quarter goal and find yourself going into quarter 2 with a 30 pound loss (losing 10 lbs a month is totally doable if you have 100 lbs to lose), you may want to revise that one year goal to be 80 or 90 pounds instead of the original 60. Then adjust the upcoming quarter accordingly.

I would suggest that you plan regular goal review periods. Definitely do a check-in at your 6 month mark, but you can also take this opportunity when you create your quarterly goals and again with each monthly goal that you set.

For many of us, failure to lose weight has resulted from a lack of flexibility with ourselves. I know that I would tend to look at my current plan or diet as an "all or nothing" type of venture. I really didn't allow much for the unknown or necessary revision and the result was often the feeling of having to "start over".

Keep in mind that this plan you've created will shift and change. It is not meant to be a "diet" that you go on or off. It is meant to keep your momentum going forward with the goal of weight loss and health long term. It is meant to create true change and a healthy lifestyle for yourself for the rest of your life.

Create a Process

When it comes to planning out your goals and strategies for success, make it fun!

In fact, I would suggest that you attach this process to something that you love. Perhaps your planning sessions can be done at your favorite local coffee shop, out to lunch at a favorite restaurant or sitting in a park by the beach.

As you start to see success along the way, you'll becomes even more motivated and excited to have these little planning meetings with yourself.

Treat them as critical…a meeting that you can't put off. Put yourself first when it comes to planing the strategy for changing your life.

If you can manage the time and the expense, I would suggest that you book yourself into a nice hotel or B&B when you set out to first create your plan. This can be a wonderful way to mark the beginning of something new and exciting in your life…to mark the day that you decided that you would create a change in your life.

Of course, you can just as well create a little mini retreat for yourself at home. If you have a family, this may require some outside support. Do this for yourself and for your family. Make yourself a priority and figure out how to put your health first on a consistent basis.

Plan Your Rewards

This part of the planning process is REALLY fun!

How and when do you want to reward yourself? This can vary depending on the things that you love and perhaps your financial situation if those things also have a monetary cost attached to them. (but they don't have to)

Begin with your ultimate reward ideas. How will you celebrate when you reach that ultimate goal? I love to travel, so for me I can imagine booking a fantastic biking trip in Italy as the perfect way to celebrate my new healthy fitness level and my love for all things Italian.

Maybe for you, it might be hiring a personal shopper and creating that awesome work wardrobe to go with your new smaller size.

Another idea might be a complete makeover - the hair cut, color, make-up - everything you can think of to celebrate your new attitude and style.

I would also suggest that you create a set of milestones that are significant to you and plan to celebrate each of them in a way that makes you feel great about the accomplishment. When you are just beginning, your first milestone may be completing all of your goals (sticking to it) for your first week. How can you reward yourself for that? At least in the beginning, I would choose something that is not food related, although I do think it is OK to treat yourself later on if you think you can do so without setting a downward trend in motion.

Other milestones might include your first 5 and 10 lbs lost. You may want to reward yourself for some fitness goal that you are working towards such as walking or riding your bike for x number of miles.

This part of the planning should be fun! You can choose big rewards or smaller things like getting a mani/pedi, buying a new candle or lotion or maybe seeing that new movie that you've been dying to see. Figure out the rewards that have meaning for you and have fun with this part of the planning.

Resources and Apps

Books About Goal Setting:

Brian Tracy

Goals!: How to Get Everything You Want -- Faster Than You Ever Thought Possible
http://www.amazon.com/dp/1605094110/

Focal Point: A Proven System to Simplify Your Life, Double Your Productivity, and Achieve All Your Goals
http://www.amazon.com/dp/0814472788/

Apps:

There are many apps available for use on your smartphone or computer than can make the process of goal tracking so easy and fun. Here are some that I would suggest you look at if you have an interest in this.

2Do

My number one planning tool that I absolutely love is an this app on my iPhone. It is visually appealing and you can create different tabs for topics that are color coded. The app has many features that I love and I use a style where I put tasks or goals within the different tabs or folders and then assign them to dates on a weekly or daily basis. For ex, I have one tab color coded for exercise. Here I have my various exercise goals for the week that I can then assign to a date.

2doapp.com

Joe's Goals

This is a simple online tool to help you check off your daily goals.

joesgoals.com

43Things

This is an online goal setting and tracking tool with the added social element. You can find goal ideas as well as other people that are working to accomplish similar goals.

43things.com

Toodledo

This is a robust online tracking and organizational system that can also integrate with a mobile phone app.

toodledo.com

Lifetick

This is an online tool that also has an app for the smart phone. This tool will allow you to create and track goals and also journal your progress.

lifetick.com

TraxItAll

This is a simple iPhone app that allows you to create and track your goals.

traxitall.com

Book 4: Eating for Weight Loss

A Note from Paula...

This volume and the next one in the series on exercise is where we will be getting into the nuts and bolts of losing weight.

Whether you're trying to lose 100+ pounds like I am, or any amount of weight, you've probably already tried a number of different diets and approaches that promise results. We all know that many of these are fad diets that aren't necessarily healthy and some of them do work and are fine for you.

As I've said before, I don't advocate any one plan or method for losing weight. I do advocate being smart and always keeping your health in mind. This means that if it sounds too good to be true, it probably isn't the healthiest method for you.

When I started on my journey to losing over 100+ pounds, I knew that the eating part of the process had to be something that I could live with long-term. I knew this was not going to be fast if I also wanted to be healthy. For me this did mean a pretty drastic change in my diet, but it also meant that no particular food would ever be off limits. I had failed in the past when I had tried to completely eliminate certain foods altogether and I needed something that would keep me moving forward with weight loss in a way that was fun and didn't leave me feeling deprived.

For me, the perfect solution was going back to the basics of calories counting on a daily or weekly basis. For the most part, this is what I will be sharing with you in this book.

In Book 4, I'd like to share with you what has worked for me in terms of the kinds of foods and menu planning that has also been completely doable and enjoyable.

This section is meant to be a blueprint to help you to develop a strategy for what you will be eating while on your journey to losing weight and changing your life.

To YOUR success,

Paula

Options for Eating to Lose Weight

Here I will briefly go over some of the main programs or methods that people choose when it comes to the food plan for losing weight. As I said earlier, I choose to count my calories and this will be the main focus of the remainder of this book, but I did want to go over a few options with you here in case you are drawn to another method. The following are in no particular order and are not personally endorsed by me. You can find links to each program website under the Resources and Apps section of the book.

Programs that Include Packaged Foods

There are some diet plans that include pre-packaged food. A few of the more popular programs would be NutriSystem and Jenny Craig, but there are others as well. For someone who is very busy and doesn't want to deal with counting calories or portion control, this type of plan can be ideal. Someone might also choose this convenience as a way to jump-start their efforts and then transition on to a more hands on approach to food preparation.

Shakes or Protein Drinks

There are diet plans that you can follow that include purchasing some shakes or drinks that can either be replacement meals or supplements to a healthy diet. Using something like Slim-Fast, for example, can also be a good option for someone who is very busy. This could be a great starting point for the person who might need some fast nutrition on the go. There are other protein drink option out there as well. Be sure to explore the complete program to know that you are getting the proper nutrition and I would recommend that these types of shakes do not comprise the bulk of your whole eating plan.

Low Carb Diet Plans (and/or High Protein Diets)

There are several popular diet plans that fit into the category of low-carb or high protein diets or a combination of the two. Some that you might recognize and wish to explore further would be the Atkins Diet, the Zone Diet and the South Beach Diet.

Programs that Look Great to Me!

Though I haven't been on a paid program during this last period of weight loss, I have done Weight Watchers in the past and I do think this is a very effective and healthy program. I especially like it because it seems very doable and is not as restrictive in the types of foods you can eat while on the plan. I've not tried the Biggest Loser Club, but being a big fan of the TV show and seeing what others have to say, this seems like another very realistic and healthy program. I also love that both of these options have a strong online community which makes it doable for even the busiest of people.

Counting Calories

We'll be talking about this method throughout the remainder of the book as this is the option I've chosen to follow on my own journey to lose over 100 pounds. Of course, ultimately any diet or program you choose basically will come down to the amount of calories you consume as compared to the amount of calories you burn. I chose to arm myself with some tools and books and take on the challenge of tracking calories for myself. Throughout this book it is my intention to give you the information and resource recommendations so that you can also lose your weight by counting calories on a daily or weekly basis.

Let's get started!

Back to Basics

If you've been struggling with your weight for a time, I'm sure you can relate to how I've felt when it comes to trying a new diet plan or the latest fast weight loss promise. I had become so fed up with starting a diet, starving myself for a period of time, eating foods that I really wasn't enjoying and then ending up with a weight gain once I realized that I couldn't stick to the program at all.

I was SO frustrated and depressed about the whole cycle of dieting. I knew yo-yo dieting wasn't healthy and I also knew I had a hard time sticking to any one plan over a long period of time.

When I made the decision to lose over 100 pounds I also knew that something had to be really different this time when it came down to what I was eating and not eating. Let's be honest, the idea of giving up my favorite foods meant nothing fun or exciting to me. Of course I knew that I needed to drastically change my daily diet, but I also determined that I wouldn't put certain foods on a complete restriction.

After some thought and research, I decided that the best way to incorporate all of the foods that I really didn't want to give up within a new healthier eating plan would be to track my calories on a regular basis. Focusing on the number of calories meant that I could "fit in" certain foods on certain days. This seemed completely doable to me and as I've already confessed in my previous book on goal setting, I can be a bit of a nerd when it comes to planning and tracking so this really seemed to suit my personality.

I call this section "Back to Basics" because I decided there was so much information out there about good foods/bad foods, good fats/bad fats, good carbs/bad carbs, etc that it was overwhelming to sort out the actual correct method for what a healthy diet actually looked like these days.

Let me take a minute to remind you that I am not a nutritionist or certified in any way to give advice that is based on any type of medical knowledge or even thoroughly researched data. You can choose to research that for yourself if you like. I consider myself to be pretty logical and at least somewhat intelligent so I just decided to go back to the basics of what I had learned in grade school regarding healthy eating and also to trust my gut in this process.

I do think as you go, you will do more research for yourself, and you may very well find yourself drawn to a diet that includes less meat or carbs for example. For me, this was about finding a starting point that also included the occasional slice of pizza when I felt it necessary.

So the basics of my diet plan included the following:

— determine my target daily calories (I will go over this more in the next section)
— a well rounded diet that consisted of lots of fruits and veggies
— paying more attention to portion sizes
— as much as possible a typical meal would consist of a large amount of veggies, regular portion of carbs, and a regular portion of lean protein
— not skimping on a snack if I was hungry in between meals (often choose fruit or a protein for my snack)
— recognizing that I had a sweet tooth during the evening and making a plan for this that would allow me to stay on track with my daily calories
— recognizing that my new calorie/eating plan was to be a work in progress - I was in this for the long haul with the goal of going only in one direction with my weight

In the next section, I'll cover some ideas for how you can determine the best calorie target for yourself and begin your planning process.

Counting Calories

We'll begin here by just covering the very basics about calories in terms of losing weight.

We've gained our weight over time by consuming more calories than what our bodies have been burning. I can tell you from experience, in my case choosing to eat fast food sometimes twice a day while maintaining a relatively sedentary lifestyle was probably easily packing on an additional few thousand calories a day. Given that 3,500 calories equals one pound, its easy to see how this could quickly add up to the added 5 pounds on a pretty regular basis.

So in order to now get this weight off, we need to create a calorie deficit on a regular basis. We can do this by decreasing the amount of calories we consume, by increasing the amount of calories we burn or a combination of the two which of course is recommended for optimal health.

I think a healthy weekly weight loss would be 1-3 lbs depending on what your starting point it. Realistically, if you have a lot of weight to lose as I did, you'll most likely lose much more than this at the beginning, but it's important to set realistic goals for yourself and to realize that it is not a process that is going to happen overnight. You will get there and you will feel better as you go way before you achieve your ultimate weight loss goal.

As noted in my earlier book, "Goal Setting for Weight Loss", when I was getting started I took the approach of adding new things to my daily/weekly routine that encompassed both the food and the exercise. I did this in a rather systematic way and in a way that was completely doable for me and this is what I would suggest to you also if you are going to drastically be changing your habits. You can take small steps that will lead to massive momentum and big results over time.

In terms of setting your first target calorie range, if you have a lot of weight to lose you might be surprised at how big this number actually could be in the beginning. I will include a link to a tool and additional resources in the resource section, but to give you an idea, when I first started at 270+ lbs, I basically multiplied my current weight by 9 (later by 7 or using an online tool) which gave me a range of about 2,400 calories/day. I was also walking and doing some other exercise and it was enough to get the weight started in the right direction.

A typical calorie target for someone who doesn't have quite the much weight to lose, might be more in the range of 1600-1800 calories/day. I would say that unless you are down to your last 10-20 pounds, most people who are at least moderately active can lose weight eating that amount of calories. There is a link to a tool in the resource section that can be useful in helping you to figure out your own calorie target.

Keep in mind that this can vary depending on what your own needs and level of activity might be. I also like to think of it as a somewhat moving target, meaning if I have days with a lot of exercise, I will definitely bump that number up a bit especially if I am hungrier than normal. I would also suggest that regardless of your weight, for women you shouldn't really be consuming less than 1200 calories a day. (more for men) I don't particularly think that a lesser number is healthy. Keep in mind that you should always consult with your own doctor as this is not meant to be medical advice.

You also might want to have an idea of what your daily target is, but really having a weekly calorie goal. This is good for someone who may need more flexibility from day to day in terms of their planning and calorie count. For example, if you have to eat out a bit for work and you think these times might result in going over a daily calorie target, you can look at it more over the course of the week and adjust your daily to allow for these occasions.

I will also talk a bit later about calorie cycling which is another way you might like to approach your calorie targets.

The most important thing when you are just getting started, is to have a calorie number that is doable and one that you can feel confident about hitting. Each week of hitting your target will bring about more and more momentum. Particularly if you are starting with a lot of weight to lose you will probably see some pretty fast weight loss as a result of your efforts.

Next we'll talk about food and how to design a food plan that will work for you..

Designing Your Food Plan

Next, we're going to talk about how to begin to design your menu and think about the types of foods you want to include as you get started on your weight loss plan.

You don't have to be a great chef or have any special knowledge about cooking in order to create meals that are healthy and enjoyable to eat. If you have little cooking experience or knowledge about general nutrition, you might want to invest in a few books or do some research online. I was definitely not a great cook when I started but I did come to enjoy cooking and developing a few favorite meals that I love to prepare on an almost weekly basis.

Firstly, I do want to say that I don't advocate cutting your favorite foods out altogether, but only you know how much you can handle if you do seem to have certain foods or meals that trigger a downward spiral. If this is the case for you, I would start out with some type of commitment in terms of abstaining from a particular food. For myself, I did choose to draw a strong line when it came to eating out for the first month or so and I think it was a good idea. I knew that eating fast food and restaurant food in general had the potential to derail me and I wanted to develop some strength during this time and allow myself to lose those first 15-20 lbs before I did choose to eat out at all.

I would start by creating lists of all your favorite foods. Any of your favorite meals can most likely be made more calorie friendly or fit into your menu planning in some way so think of the things that you really love to eat.

One example for myself that seemed to be a nice treat was a burger and fries dinner. I do this meal on a regular basis and it totally feels like a treat. Here is what that meal consists of and looks like in terms of calories - turkey patty (Jennie-O, frozen), 2 pieces of wheat bread toasted, slice of kraft cheese, pickles, 2 servings of Ore-Ida French Fries (cooked in the oven), ketchup and Ranch dressing. All of this comes to roughly 635 calories and it could be done with less. I don't do this every evening but I can plan for it if I feel like I need/want it and its totally doable within my calories for a day/week.

Another example of something I love (and maybe you do too) is pizza. I will have on occasion (usually once/week) 1/2 of a frozen 4 meat Tombstone pizza with a large salad and Ranch dressing. The 1/2 pizza is 750 calories which is a bit on the high side for a meal, but my point is that if you know you can work these items into your regular eating you'll be much less likely to splurge outside of your plan and you can feel completely satisfied. This would be a meal I would typically have after my weigh-in day for the week as an example. I would eat 1/2 one day and the other 1/2 the next.

Now I did start out here with a few higher calorie examples because I really want to stress to you that this is about creating a plan that will work for YOU. It is not about giving up everything you love at all. I really want you to get the sense that you will be developing better and healthier eating habits but it doesn't mean that you won't be able to eat your favorite meals, even while you are on this weight loss journey. This is NOT about going on a diet that you will then go off of at some later date in the future - even after you reach your goal weight. This is about changing your life for the long term and developing habits that you will be able to live with for the rest of your life.

So here I just want you to work on your favorite food lists and think about some ways that you might make some substitutions to make those meals more calorie friendly for you. You could even plan out your weekly menu and purposefully include some of these favorite meals for your very first week. This may prove to you that if you are diligent in your tracking and resolve, you can lose weight eating the foods that you love and will get you off to the very best start.

In the next section, I'll share with you my typical food lists and meals so that you can get some ideas and also see that there is nothing ultra fancy about what I am eating. You can probably be way more fancy than I am!

Meal and Snack Ideas

Here I will lay out some typical meals that I might have along with an approximate calorie count. This is not meant to be specific - you will be looking at particular calorie information for the various foods that you'll be putting together, but this is to give you an idea of all the foods that I do enjoy on a regular basis.

Breakfast Ideas

I always start my day with 2-3 cups of coffee and I would be using either skim milk or low-fat half-n-half so the calories for this would vary from about 36-60 calories.

2 pieces of low calorie wheat toast
peanut butter
banana (yes I make a sandwich with this!)
275 calories

2 scrambled eggs with ham and low fat cheese
2 pieces of wheat toast with Margarine
390 calories

2 frozen waffles
banana or berries
low sugar syrup
270 calories

2 pancakes (I love Fiber One mix)
banana or berries
low sugar syrup
310 calories

1.5 serving of oatmeal with brown sugar
banana or berries
1/2 cup skim milk
410 calories

Other things I might have include various cereal with fruit or maybe a smoothie made with juice and frozen fruit. I don't care for yogurt myself, but this is a great option for getting some protein with your breakfast meal.

I never skip breakfast (or any meal for that matter) and find that eating a healthy meal in the morning can help to set the tone for a good day.

Lunch Ideas (most of these will be 300-500 calories)

Typically for lunch I might have leftovers from my dinner the night before. As a single person, I rarely cook only one portion for this reason. If I am making a dinner with chicken, rice and peanut sauce for example. I will cook 3 portions of the chicken so that I can use 2 portions with a lunch salad during the week. Or I might cook 2 portions of the chicken with rice so that I can have one of those for lunch the next day. A little organization here goes a long way towards your success when it comes to meal planning.

BIG salads
— I do not use portion control when it comes to lettuce and most veggies. I say take a big bowl and fill it with greens - the greener the better. Choose whatever you fancy for your salad. It's great to get a nice serving of protein in there. I especially like chicken with some Parmesan cheese, but you could choose other proteins such as ham, steak or hard boiled eggs. Another example of what I would do is to cook 2 portions of beef taco meat for dinner one night and use the second portion the next day to make a yummy taco salad with Ranch dressing and salsa.

— This is a great opportunity to experiment with some vegetables if you are not used to eating them. I like to use different colored bell peppers, green onions, cucumbers, etc. You'll find yourself feeling a very healthy type of full after eating a nice big salad for lunch.

— Of course the main key to keeping the calorie count reasonable for your salad is the type of dressing you choose. I like many of the Kraft Lite dressings…especially the Asian (with my peanut sauced chicken) and the different vinaigrettes. I also do admit to loving Ranch dressing on the side of things like fries and pizza as well as on some of my salads, so I also always keep a big bottle of the Kraft Light Ranch. (personally I don't like the taste of the fat free dressings, so I always opt for the low fat versions) Also be very careful not to overdue the serving when it comes to dressing your salad.

— If I am having my favorite big chicken salad with peanut sauce and Asian dressing (I include some lite Mandarin oranges with this salad), I might also have a small flour tortilla on the side. I like to start by making a little wrap with a bunch of the salad inside.

Soup and Sandwich
— I love the Healthy Choice canned soups and will often heat up a whole can (2 servings) for lunch and have it with a grilled cheese sandwich.

Quesadilla with cheese and chicken if I have some (or sometimes I do sausage and cheese with Ranch dressing on the side) with lots of salsa

So for lunch, most of the time it would be something listed above or a left-over portion of the dinner meals that you will see below.

Dinner Ideas (most of these will be 500-700 calories)

Pasta with beef sauce
Parmesan cheese
salad with Ranch dressing
— I will cook a lb of beef and then put it in a jar of plain or garlic tomato pasta sauce.
—Typically I will also freeze the beef sauce in 2 serving portions as it is very easy to heat up and makes for a quick dinner.

Pasta with Pesto, sausage and sundried tomatoes
Parmesan cheeses
salad with Vinaigrette dressing
— I make the Pesto with 2 seasoning packets. (I do use less of the called for Olive Oil, substituting with a greater portion of water)
— I portion these into ice cube trays and freeze them - once frozen I put them in a Freezer Zip-lock bag and each cube is about 35 calories.
— This is another very easy thing to do with Pasta - just pop a few of the cubes into the microwave and coat your past with the Pesto.
— Of course you could do the same with homemade Pesto which would be even better.

Chicken with some type of sauce - I love to just buy a bottled Peanut Sauce as well as some of the other spicier types of sauces.
I love to eat this mixed right in with Basmati rice usually.
You can also throw in come green beans, brocolli or other veggie with this rice dish.

Beef Tacos (I just use the Taco Bell seasoning packet - see, I told you it wasn't too fancy!)
2 small flour tortillas
low fat Mexican cheese
salsa
Ranch

Baked Fish (I like Tilapia)
— I coat the fish with bread crumbs, Old Bay seasoning and a dash of Pam spray before putting it in the oven.
— Once cooked I put lemon juice, capers and some Parmesan cheese on top.
— Depending on what else I am having with this meal, I might also have some tartar sauce as the calories are reasonable if you watch the portion.
— I like to eat this fish with either Angel Hair pasta and pesto or homemade mashed potatoes with garlic.
— I would also have a salad or some other type of veggies with this - Asparagus is a great option.

Homemade Mac-n-Cheese

— This can be a great comfort food option if you're in the mood - the key is portion control.

— I use elbow macaroni, 1 Tb or so of real butter, low fat Mexican cheese with Parmesan on top.

— I sometimes like to do this with sausage or ham.

— Salad on the side is great for this.

As mentioned earlier, I also do frozen pizza and turkey burgers and fries on occasion.

Snacks and Sweet Ideas

Typically I have 2-3 snacks throughout the day. Usually I have a late morning snack, a late afternoon snack and some type of sweet after dinner.

These can range from 100 calories or less to 300 or so, depending on how much exercise I am doing on a given day.

Below are items that I will typically have for a snack - in some cases it will be combo of 2 items.

— piece of fruit - banana, apple, orange, kiwi, etc
— low fat string cheese
— hard boiled egg
— toast with peanut butter or jam
— crackers
— pretzels
— hummus
— veggies - carrots, celery, cucumber, etc
— 1 small tortilla with cheese and salsa
— small bowl of cereal
— fruit smoothie

Here are some sweets I like to have in the evening.

— low fat vanilla ice cream (I often make a float with Diet A&W
Root Beer - yummy!)
   — any of the 100 calories sweets or snacks
   — low fat graham crackers
   — sugar free jello with low fat Cool Whip
   — low fat puddings

This is just meant to give you some ideas so that you know that
I've not been eating any special "diet foods" on my weight loss plan.
Design a menu that works for you and is somewhat varied if you think
this will help you to succeed.

Next, we'll talk about the importance of tracking your food and
calories.

Importance of Tracking

Once of the most critical pieces of being successful when it comes to counting calories will be the accuracy of which you measure and track the food and calories that you are consuming.

In the beginning, this may seem to be a bit of a chore as you will constantly be looking up calorie counts and measuring your ingredients and items, but trust me when I say that this will get much easier and faster as you go along.

Also there are great tracking tools that you can use online or on your smartphone that will make this part of the process a lot easier. When I started I did record everything with a calorie counting book or looking it up online and then reporting it in my notebook. These days I use an app on my iPhone that I love and makes the process so much easier. I will include that in the resource section so that you can check it out for yourself.

One of the reasons that I know I put on so much weight over the years was that I spent a significant amount of time not paying much attention or even being in denial about how much food I was actually consuming.

This process will help you to get back on track with knowing what you are eating and also help you to be more accountable when it comes to how much you are eating.

Truly the first step for many of us, is just getting out of that denial so this is a step that is critical.

As you go, you'll find that it will become easier to eyeball measurements and you'll also get to know what the calorie count of certain foods are.

Next, we'll talk about an area of frustration for many people…the dreaded plateau ad how you may be able to combat that with something known as calorie cycling.

Using Calorie Cycling to Break a Plateau

Calorie cycling is also called zig-zag dieting or calorie shifting. It is a method of calorie counting that has been known to help you break out of a plateau period.

Over time with your weight loss, you will most likely experience the dreaded plateau. This is when you can be doing the exact same things in terms of eating and exercise and your scale just does not seem to want to move. This can be very frustrating if a pound loss is important to you.

One option for breaking a plateau is doing calorie cycling for a period of time and this can also be something you might want to use to shake up your routine a bit.

Calorie cycling is a method where you have a weekly calorie target as opposed to a consistent daily target. The idea behind this is that having some variation or extremes with your daily calorie intake will "trick" your metabolism and get your weight loss going again.

For example, you may have 2 days in a row that are normal at 1600 calorie targets and then a 2000 calorie target followed by another day with a 1300 calorie target.

In my experience, this method does work for breaking a plateau which can be extremely frustrating. I have also used this method when I know that I will be having a few higher calorie days due to eating out or something out of the ordinary.

I will include a link in the resource section to an online tool that can help you to figure out a week of calorie cycling targets for you according to your current weight and activity level.

Yes, You CAN Have Taco Bell

I believe that much of my 140 lb weight gain was due to eating fast food. Taco Bell, McDonalds, Burger King, Pizza Hut…the list goes on and on.

Confession time: At the peak of my self-sabotage, I would go through multiple drive-thrus to get exactly the food I was craving - rush home, sit in front of the TV and devour the food…stuff, stuff, stuff myself until I had that weird satisfied (full!) feeling. I hated myself at those times but in the moment it was the only thing that I thought would make me feel better. (OK, consciously I may not even have been thinking about it at all…habits can be SO powerful)

Today I no longer feel the need to do multiple drive-thru runs but I do sometimes allow myself a bit of fast food or whatever it is I may be craving.

Before beginning my weight loss, I had tried to diet many times and I really believe that my all-or-nothing mentality is part of what led to failure during those attempts. When I set out to lose the weight this final time, I vowed to be more realistic with myself. Yes, I wanted to add good healthy foods to my diet BUT I really didn't want to say goodbye to my favorite junk foods forever.

I did know starting out that for me I needed a period of time though when I would be very strict on myself with the dieting…I didn't want to chance the pull of the habit. So I did give up all eating out for the first month or so. The more times I said no to my cravings during this time, the stronger I became. You'll get there too, I promise.

Over time, I've discovered that I really can have pretty much what I want and am craving, not allowing myself to go crazy or anything.

If I'm sticking with my exercise for the week/month and eating healthy choices 80-90% of the time, I really do find that if I'm having a particular craving one day I can plan for that meal and be perfectly fine.

Here are some planning suggestions based on calorie counting:

1. Know what you are going to order and what the calorie count will be. (roughly) Guess what? Taco Bell has their full menu online with all of the nutritional information. I wanted to have 2 Volcano Burritos (I know disgusting! lol), but since those babies were 800 calories a pop, I settled for 2 chicken soft tacos and 1 regular/beef soft taco - calories count 610…not bad and totally doable. (NOW if I had decided to have the 2 Volcanoes - which I might do on a given day, I'd try to eat 1200-1300 calories most days of that same week and definitely not fore-go the exercise!)

2. Plan your calories for the rest of the day. A big calorie meal out may require that you adjust your calories for the rest of the day. Know what you'll be having for the other 2-3 meals throughout the day.

3. Exercise! Exercise! Exercise! Don't feel bad after you eat that pizza once a month that you've been craving! Commit to an extra great cardio day before, of and after! No sweat! No guilt! Trade for it! It's allowed.

4. No guilt! Vow to enjoy the meal that you've planned for. Guilt is NOT necessary here. Do you know why? Because you are conscious…not eating on autopilot. You've made the decision to indulge and tomorrow you will make the decision to be completely on your healthy track.

I'm really trying to keep it real here with you…hope you know that! I've been known to eat a small pizza and chicken wings (all of them!) on the 1st of the month after a successful weigh-in…and the next day, I get up do my cardio and plan a salad for lunch!

Enter the no guilt zone and enjoy!

Enjoying the Holidays or Special Events

I wanted to be sure to include some suggestions about how to deal with meals and indulgences over the holiday season or special events, because I know that this can be something that a lot of us struggle with and I don't want it to derail you from your good efforts. I think many of us equate the holidays with big meals and weight gain. With a bit of planning and consciousness though, there's no reason not to be able to enjoy a great meal and either not lose weight or have a very quick recovery after gaining a few pounds.

Here are some tips that might help. Remember, planning is the key to navigating all of these challenges during your weight loss journey!

1. Have a rough idea (unless you are cooking, in which case you will know) of what food will be served.

For our example here we'll choose the Thanksgiving meal. We can pretty much bet on the traditional turkey with all the fix-ins that come along with it. Pumpkin pie is my absolute favorite! (for my reader not in the US, think about your Christmas dinner or equivalent big meal with traditional food items)

2. Plan to be diligent with your meals the week of the big meal.

In the case of Thanksgiving for example, I would be planning low calorie days (for me this might look like 1200-1400 calories) Mon-Wed that week. I'd be sure to drink all my water and most likely big salads will be on the menu for lunches. Mind you, we're still being healthy here. We're not starving ourselves on these days, BUT any thoughts of pizza or dessert will be pushed back with the reminder of the Thursday meal ahead.

3. Plan to be diligent with your exercise the week of the big meal.

Make your exercise plan for the week and stick to it! It may also be a great idea to plan a little extra. I know one year on Thanksgiving, I enjoyed a wonderful (and long) morning bike ride the day of Thanksgiving. I was able to think about how thankful I was in regards to my health and how far I had come in my weight loss journey.

4. Don't go "unconscious" while you are eating the big meal.

Sit at the table with the intention to be present while you are eating. Personally, I think you should eat what you like at special occasions such as this, BUT keep portion control in mind and be conscious of eating to the point of satisfaction and not until you are feeling so stuffed that you can hardly get up from the table. Save room for that piece of pumpkin pie or the dessert that you have your eye on. Enjoy the company.

5. The day and week after, get right back into your routine!

Plan to get right back to it the next day. If you're the one cooking, give away your left-overs. If not, accept only turkey which would be great in a sandwich or on your nice big salad the next day. Do not use this meal as a complete deviation from your weight loss plan. You can eat this meal on Thursday, be back to routine on Friday and not have gained any weight (maybe even lost lbs) by Monday. Trust me, this can happen AND you can enjoy the meal and indulge just a bit.

I think too often we just equate the holidays with weight gain and accept defeat in this area and there is absolutely no reason to have this mentality. Your weight loss challenge is all about small changes that have big effects in the long run of your life. Planning for the holiday meals is just one of those life events that will keep on coming. And if you do gain 5 lbs, it's not the end of the world. You know how to lose it, and the key will be losing those 5 lbs right away and not going the other direction, using it as an excuse to gain another 5 lbs.

Let the festivities begin!

Giving Yourself a Break

I definitely want to encourage you to NOT beat yourself up if you miss a calorie target or "mess up" on a given day with your food choices.

I truly believe THE most important thing with an occasion such as this is how you handle the next day.

I believe that in most of the case when we "go off a diet" and fail, it's because we don't really give ourselves permission to get right back on track. Most of the time, one unexpected detour can lead to a complete derailment of our plan if we don't remain conscious of what we are doing and what our long term goals are.

I say that you should definitely give yourself a break, cut yourself some slack and PLAN for some special occasion "treat days".

I am not exaggerating when I say that one of the days that I always look forward to is the day after a successful monthly weigh-in. It is typically a time for pizza (small) and chicken wings and you better believe that I look forward to and enjoy every last lick off my fingers.

It really is time to give yourself a break from all of the negative self talk and behavior patterns that have been leading you to a place where you don't feel proud or good about yourself.

You really can get this food plan under your control in a way that doesn't leave you feeling deprived and will lead to your weight loss and forward momentum.

You can do this!

Resources and Apps

Programs and Diet Plans Mentioned in the Options for Eating to Lose Weight Section:

nutrisystem.com
jennycraig.com
slim-fast.com
atkins.com
zonediet.com
southbeachdiet.com
weightwatchers.com
biggestloserclub.com

Calorie Counting Books:

The Biggest Loser Calorie Counter
http://www.amazon.com/dp/1594865957/

The CalorieKing Calorie, Fat, & Carbohydrate Counter 2012
http://www.amazon.com/dp/1930448368/

The Calorie Counter For Dummies
http://www.amazon.com/dp/0470568348/

Websites and Useful Tools:

Fitwatch

This website has some very good information and tools to do with calorie counting.

fitwatch.com

Calorie Cycling:

Here is a website and tool that will help you to figure out a good calorie cycling plan.

freedieting.com/tools/calorie_calculator.htm

Apps:

There are many apps available for use on your smartphone or computer than can make the process of tracking calories easier. Here are some that I would suggest you look at if you have an interest in this.

Lose It

This is the app that I am currently using on my iPhone to track my calories on a daily and weekly basis. It is easy to use and allows for adding your own foods to the database. You can also track your exercise with this app although I am not currently using this feature.

loseit.com

My Plate Calorie Tracker

This is another app that will allow you to track your daily calories. It has been developed by Livestrong.com.

livestrong.com/thedailyplate/iphone-calorie-tracker/

Calorie Counter & Diet Tracker by MyFitnessPal

This is another popular calorie tracking app for the iPhone.

myfitnesspal.com/iphone

Book 5: Exercise for Weight Loss

A Note from Paula…

This volume and the last one in the series on eating is where we are getting into the nuts and bolts of losing weight…meaning dealing with the calories we put into our bodies and the calories that we will burn to get the weight off.

If you have a significant amount of weight to lose as I did, you're probably not really excited about the exercise piece. I was severely overweight and couldn't bear the thought of walking more than 15 minutes, let along hitting the local gym where everyone could see my 270+ lb body on the treadmill. (Hint, people don't really care all that much, but I get why you might feel intimidated - I did too)

Listen. I SO get where you are at if that's you. I could barely walk up the 2 flights of stairs to my apartment building without feeling winded so it was difficult for me to get behind a significant exercise program. This idea really goes back to what I said about starting where you are in the book about goal setting. I really mean that. Don't make it big and scary right now. This whole process of getting the weight off is a journey. It won't happen all at once, BUT it will happen and get easier if you make this process about realistic stepping stones.

You DON'T have to join the local gym and commit to an hour of cardio right now if your body and mind are not at that place yet.

What you do need to do is start moving MORE…more than what you did last week and you will do much more next month than you will be doing this week.

I promise you it will get easier. Your body will adjust to working out and it will start to feel good.

The weight will start to come off and you'll notice that you feel lighter when you are working out.

You'll be going along developing some great workout habits and one day 6 months from now when you are down 40-60 lbs, you'll catch a glimpse of yourself in the mirror and be overcome with a feeling of pride and anticipation for the changes you have made and the one direction you are now headed.

You will feel strong in your body as you go about your day, feeling more and more confident about the new habits and changes you are making in your own life.

In Book 5, I'd like to share with you what has worked for me in terms of exercise and help you with some ideas that are completely doable and enjoyable for you.

This section is meant to be a blueprint to help you to develop a realistic and fun exercise plan that will help you to burn calories and get your body in shape.

To YOUR success,

Paula

Why You Should Exercise

You are probably well aware of the knowledge that you "should" be exercising. There are so many reasons to do it. The fact that we haven't been doing it has greatly led to our weight gain. I can speak for myself here because at 278 lbs, I was not exercising at all. I was working from home sitting in front of my computer which was greatly contributing to what had become a very sedentary lifestyle.

There are many reasons why one should exercise, even for people who are not overweight. I'm not going to get into all of the technical bits and pieces of this - you can find loads of books and materials online about how exercise effects the body. I am going to speak to the benefits I have personally gained from exercising. I am guessing that if you are coming from a place similar to where I was with 100+ lbs to lose and feeling depressed, you will also notice many of these benefits. Please trust me as you begin your own exercise plan.

Here are some of the many benefits that I received from exercising even long before I lost a significant amount of weight. As I am writing these, I'm specifically thinking about my walks and long bike rides, but imagine doing the things that you love in terms of your own program that you will design.

Fresh air

This might seem obvious, but as someone who was very obese and also working from home I really had to make a point of getting outside during the day. Once I started my workout routine I would actually prefer to break it up into smaller time periods so that I had a chance to get up from my computer and get outside for some fresh air.

Help with depression

At 278 pounds, I was dealing with some depression. Quite frankly I think it's hard not to be somewhat depressed at that size. Of course I believe that the inside is more important than the outside, that you can still be heavy and be beautiful...all of that and I know some people might take offense to the comment. All I can say from my own experience is that it's hard to imagine feeling physically good enough at that size to the point where your physical aches and discomforts don't affect your mood and emotional outlook. I know for me this was true and I just felt down about it.

I had thought about going to a doctor to possibly get on some medication but the depression was mild enough that I really believed it was situational and that it would lift as soon as I was feeling better about my body and losing some of the weight. What I didn't really expect was that I started feeling much better emotionally way before I really got any significant weight off. I definitely attribute this to exercise, eating better and the good feelings that came from achieving my daily and weekly goals consistently.

Get in touch with your body

In the earlier book on motivation, I talked about how out of touch we get with our bodies when we are heavy. Really I would go so far as to say that I could be in complete denial at times...until I caught a glance of myself in a window while shopping for example. Yikes! Part of the importance of this journey to lose the weight and change your life will be about being fully conscious in your body. You'll begin to notice true hunger, the signals of illness or injury and you will just begin to actually claim ownership of your body once again. Exercising really helped me to get in touch with that piece that had been missing for so long. Your body and the things it is capable of are glorious! Please enjoy every bit of the process of recognition as to how your body serves you and how you are now taking care of it.

Feel good about achieving your goals

I am a bit of a geek when it comes to goal setting and planning. I loved that I could set weekly goals around exercise that were first simple and completely doable and later more challenging in order to push myself. If you are not used to feeling successful about exercise, this is something that can be a fast win for you. To begin, set smaller exercise goals and then go from there. Enjoy the process of crossing one more item off your list that is contributing to your commitment to create a new life for yourself.

Time for yourself

Depending on your current family and living situation, your workouts might be an ideal time for you to really have some quiet time to yourself. Though I am single and mostly living alone, there is something about walking (or biking) by myself that really gets me into a certain zone. I can imagine that if you are a parent, wife/husband or a busy career woman/man that this might be a well deserved break from the normal daily living. Try to enjoy this time to yourself.

Time with a friend

Exercising with a buddy can also be equally as great! If you are busy and have a difficult time scheduling social activities with your friends consider inviting them to join you for a bit of exercising. Walking is perfect for this because chatting with a friend makes the time pass so quickly. It can also be a great source of support and commitment to schedule regular workouts with a friend or group of friends.

Increased creativity

I found that during my exercise time ideas would really start to flow. It seems that my creativity completely opened up to me when I was in this zone. I began to carry a notepad with me (and later just used an app on my iPhone) to capture various new ideas and ideas for projects that I currently had going.

Learn something new

I never go walking without my iPhone/iPod. Listening to various podcasts or something inspirational has been instrumental in my motivation to exercise. Sometimes I actually look forward to my walk mainly because I'm dying to listen to a new podcast or a motivational series that I am currently into. What you listen to should suit your own interests, but you can find free podcasts on almost any topic. You could also listen to your favorite music or an audiobook. If you really want to kill two birds with one stone, get a language learning program and learn that new language that you never seem to be able to find the time to start. The possibilities are endless, so make it fun for you.

Exercise will encourage the likelihood of sticking with your food plan

I really think that a regular exercise plan will also help you to stick to your food plan for a given week. After you start enjoying some of the benefits that you will feel after an exercise session, you're much less likely to give in to any fast food craving or eat things that aren't serving the new healthier you. Most likely when you start to reach your 40+ minute cardio workouts, you will feel a healthy type of hunger and start to crave foods that are good for your body.

Explore new places

I started working out after I moved across the country from California to North Carolina. I did not keep my car when I made this move, so once I bought my bicycle and starting really getting into that as my main source of exercise and transportation it allowed me to explore the city in a way that I hadn't had access to. It was fun!

Aids in weight loss

I am including the most obvious benefit of exercise here at the end because I know that for most of us, this is really the motivation to start exercising. There is no doubt that exercise will speed up any plan to lose weight. If you are watching your calories and exercising on a regular basis, the weight will come off and every drop of sweat will be worth it!

In the next section, I want to talk about a concern that I had and one that you might have also if you have a significant amount of weight to lose.

Do You Have a Fear of Loose Skin?

I definitely did when I was looking ahead at losing over 100 pounds! I had seen pictures of people who had lost similar amounts of weight and it did make me fearful because I doubted it would be any time in the near future that I could afford the surgery that would solve such an issue.

Ultimately, you'll probably come to the place that I came to which is that it's better and healthier to deal with this potential issue of loose skin than to keep unhealthy weight on our bodies.

I'm sure that this will vary from person to person and again everything I'm sharing in these books is based on only my personal experience, but there are two main factors that I believe caused me to not really have this issue.

1. I wasn't extreme with how fast I lost the weight. I do think that when people lose weight too quickly it is difficult for the body to adjust. As mentioned in the previous books, I am all about healthy weight loss. This means that it can be slow and steady and if you are also very focused on your fitness level, the process can be incredible throughout the whole journey even if you would like the weight to come off faster.

2. The other factor that I believe contributed greatly to not having loose skin is the fact that I was very conscience and methodical about how I incorporated exercise right from the beginning of my weight loss plan. I had heard from a lot of sources that one shouldn't wait to include strength training into a weight loss routine so I heeded this advice early on.

I'm not saying that you need to start lifting weights from Day 1 of your plan, but I do recommend you incorporate some gradual type of strength training into your routine as soon as you feel you are able. I think many people make the mistake of working on this piece after they have lost the weight or are far into the weight loss.

I'm not an expert at this, but I can tell you my own personal experience reflects that this can have a huge benefit when you do this early on.

I pretty much just started adding this and worked very consistently at it. Of course with much of the weight still on my body, I really couldn't notice much in terms of my muscles or how toned I was getting.

I can remember two occasions very clearly that were big Aha's to me. One was all of the sudden REALLY seeing myself in the mirror one day. I was wearing a tank top and pretty much did a double take, wondering if those were really my arms. Another time my sister was in for a visit and hadn't seen me for awhile. We were getting ready to go for a bike ride and I had a sleeveless open back top on. She about came out of her chair in shock and said she couldn't believe how toned and strong I looked from that angle.

I don't say any of this to brag and I am actually working hard now to get back to that place again but I just tell you this because it really came from small steps over time and keeping with it week after week.

I think the fact that I was doing strength training and core work along with cardio pretty much from the beginning ALONG with the fact that I was losing the weight at a very healthy pace greatly contributed to my not having a lot of loose skin after losing a great deal of weight.

I say this to encourage you and also point out that the vision you might have in your head of fit women lifting weights and looking awesome at the gym "may" have you laughing out loud at yourself at certain times when you look in the mirror while attempting this yourself. This was MY reality at 270+ lbs for sure. BUT stay with it…focus on every single good thing you are doing for yourself….focus on how strong you are getting! You will get there!

In the next section, we'll talk about the three types of exercise that you should consider incorporating into your plan.

A Three-Pronged Approach

I have learned a few things from others and reading books when it comes to losing weight and the types of exercise one should do. Of course we would all agree that some type of cardio exercise that really gets our heart rate going will be a key factor to burning calories and losing the fat. I think that a lot of people tend to put all of their focus on cardio and that this can be a mistake. I know in the past I had thought that I would add other things to my routine such as strength training AFTER I lost the weight.

Because I had heard so many times about the value in doing the strength training from the beginning, when I initially created my own plan for weight loss, I decided to take a three-pronged approach to exercise that would include the following key areas.

Cardio

This was the first thing to implement and I knew it really would be the most critical as we need to get our bodies moving to burn off the fat and lose the weight. Cardio exercise would include anything that really gets your heart rate going. This could be walking, running, biking, kick boxing, circuit training, aerobic classes, various team sports, etc. If you're just getting started and don't really have a good idea of what you will love, I suggest walking. It's fun, easy and will get you outside.

Strength Training

I have to say that out of all the things I did right with my earliest stages of implementation, choosing to start using weights earlier rather than later had to be one of the best decisions. Even though you won't be able to see those muscles for some time (under all the fat, right?), remind yourself of how strong you are getting and that you are preparing your body from the inside out. I started by doing some simple machines at my small apartment gym and then created my own routine using dumb bells and a few other items later on that I still do today.

179

Stretching and Core Work

I think this piece is critical in the beginning because like with the strength training, you are focusing on the foundation of your body. Getting your core muscle groups strong and healthy will effect everything else that you do. I also found that stretching and Pilates, which is my core exercise of choice, helped me to be more in touch with my body during the early stages.

I will go into more detail about how I personally went about incorporating these different types of exercises, but for now I just want you to have a sense of why I chose to begin with these three things in mind. I also want to stress that you will be developing your own plan, so what is fun and works for me may not feel right for you and that's OK. I just don't want you to NOT consider doing something because it is new or you think for some reason that you can't do it.

Believe me when I say that I never would have done my Pilates routines in the early days in front of anyone! Meaning, it can be rough going at the beginning but the beauty of this is the progress you will make and see as you go. THAT my friend, will be one of many wins for you along the way!

Still feeling wary about exercise? Next, we'll talk about how to find something you love. Yes, I believe that you will find something too.

Find Something You Love

If you are someone who thinks that they will never enjoy exercise, you are definitely not alone. I know that many of us look at the gym fanatics like they are crazy for being that in love with working out.

You may never get there with loving your exercise sessions and I'm here to tell you that it is really OK. You're not alone and some days will be OK and others maybe not so good when it comes to hitting the gym or your exercise goals for the week.

I'm just going to be straight with you and say that you must exercise. Learn as best you can to just suck it up and do it. Of course this assumes that you also have the go ahead from you doctor and are not experiencing a physical issue that would keep you from exercising.

You will learn to enjoy the benefits from working out and really there is nothing that will compare to how great it can make you feel, especially when you start to see the weight coming off faster as a result of increased exercise.

If you hate the idea of putting on your big sweats to exercise next to all of the hard bodies at the gym, do not start out by doing this. Although I will say that if you are interested in going to the gym, please do not let your current size or fitness level discourage you at all. You might be surprised at the support you can actually find in the gym. Most people really only care about their own workout and body so most likely if there is any judgment going on, it will be happening within your own head.

Find something you do enjoy. This is by far the best solution to getting started and it might take some hits and misses to find out what that particular thing might be for you.

I will use my own experience here as an example in the hopes that you might be able to relate to something here for yourself.

When I was just getting started with my weight loss plan, I weighed 278 lbs. I couldn't walk up a flight of stairs without feeling winded. I was getting to a point where I was having a lot of swelling in my feet and legs along with some numbness which was really starting to alarm me. I was actually concerned about exercising in general because I worried that I could have a heart attack or something and the whole idea of this was worrisome. This is one reason why I did see a doctor and want to stress that you also need to do this at the beginning to be sure of what you are physically able to do.

In the previous book on goal setting, I described how I began with a 30 day walking challenge where I committed to walking 1 hour a day for 30 days. It is not necessary to begin with a goal like this and in retrospect it probably was a bit lofty. I won't get into details, but let's just say that I could NOT walk for 60 minutes or even 30 minutes at a time. I ended up walking around my apartment complex grounds four different times throughout the day for 15 minutes at a time. That's what I could do at 278 lbs...walk for 15 minutes. AND it was hard....AND it didn't feel great the first few times...AND it did get much easier.

So, start with what you can do and preferably what you like to do.

I much prefer exercising outside to being in the gym. I always have. I also love to pair my working out with listening to one of my favorite podcasts that involve travel or online business. I think walking is a great way for anyone to begin. Once you have good shoes, there's no cost, you can do it pretty much anywhere and there is just something so motivating about being out in the fresh air.

I do like walking for sure, but now I'm going to tell you about something that completely changed how I feel about working out.

The Day I Bought a Bike

I'm not sure when I started thinking about buying a bicycle, but my first thought was that I might be too big to actually ride a bike. I believe I was about 250 lbs or so. I remember I went to the local bike shop and with hands on hips asked the sales guy if fat people could ride bikes. He looked at me and shrugged saying something to the effect of, well of course silly we sell bikes to 300+ lb men in here all the time. He was awesome actually! I told him what my main concerns were. I wanted THE most comfortable (big) seat and something that would allow me to go long distances. I left that day with my first Trek bike.

As mentioned earlier, at this time in my life I was living in North Carolina and I did not have a car. I had the bike totally geeked out with saddle bags and everything I would need to make this an actual mode of transportation.

Now mind you, I hadn't even been on a bike since I was a kid. We'll say it had been more than 20 years. For all I knew I would be the one exception to the rule about never forgetting how to ride a bike. I took the bike home and didn't really plan to get on it for a few days.

The day I took the bike out for the first time it looked like rain but I decided I would just go for a short spin around the neighborhood. I am not exaggerating when I say that being on the bicycle for the first time completely took me back to my childhood. I had found my exercise of choice. I loved it from the moment I first pedaled that day. As I was finishing the ride, it began to rain which caused me to bike as fast as I could and it did NOT feel like exercise…it was FUN!

From that moment on, I felt like I had opened the door to some special secret about exercising and weight loss. Don't get me wrong, certainly there would be days when I did not feel like getting on the bike, but once I was going it was SO wonderful. I started riding for hours at a time whenever I could. I would ride my bike to get groceries, run errands and to any appointments that I had. You know what? The weight started to come off and I felt SO fit. I would challenge myself with distance and hit a record of 50+ miles only a few months after buying my bike.

It is possible to find something you love to do. Think back to your childhood or high school days if you were involved in athletics at all. Maybe you were a runner and it wouldn't take much to get you back into that high of distance running. If you played a team sport, maybe you can get involved in a local club or get some people that you know together to take part in a game. Maybe you love to dance and the latest Zumba Dvd is calling your name.

Try a lot of things until you find the ones that feel the best to you.

If you should still hate exercise at the end of trying a bunch of new things, in a loving way I say, suck it up! It WILL get you to where you want to be! It WILL be worth it. Trust me. Trust yourself to just push through any resistance.

In the next section, we'll talk a bit about setting your goals for exercise.

Setting Realistic Exercise Goals

I go into greater detail with how to break down your goals for your weight loss plan in the earlier book on goal setting, but here I would like to give you some suggestions that are specific to your exercise goals.

Firstly if you have a lot of weight to lose and aren't used to exercising on a regular basis, the best thing you can do for yourself is to start out with goals that are completely doable. Don't get me wrong in that I don't want you to dwell here for more than your first few weeks, but I think it is important to set yourself up for success right from the beginning.

I want your first feelings of achievement just to come from keeping your promises to yourself and this includes the area of exercise.

I would suggest that you have some idea of where you are headed in terms of longer term exercise goals. I think it is better for your overall weight loss plan if you start off with the idea that you will be mixing up your various types of exercise and adding new things as you go. You'll find after a bit that some of the things you've been doing successfully to drop pounds seem to reach a level of plateau when it comes to weight loss on the scale. During times like this it can do wonders to shake up your current routine a bit.

This is one reason why I loved doing the three pronged approach to my exercise plan. When I started to lose weight pretty rapidly, for the most part I was focused on walking as my form of exercise. Gradually I would then introduce my strength training, ab work and Pilates into the mix. The fact that you don't have to start with everything will probably help you to feel less overwhelmed and it can also give you some great goals to work towards.

I want to mention that you should always schedule a visit with your doctor before you begin any type of exercise plan so please do not skip this step. You really do need to have the clean bill of health when it comes to exerting your body and getting your heart rate going.

Just to give you an idea, here is what I would suggest in terms of goals for someone who is starting at 278 lbs with little to no regular exercise currently. (this was me!) You can certainly adjust this based on your current physical capabilities, but I don't want you to overwhelm yourself right at the beginning as it can potentially end up derailing you.

For your first week on your plan, I'd suggest that your real focus is to get moving. Make the commitment to get outside and walk this first week for a minimum of three 15 minute sessions. Anything above that can be a bonus. But make a goal that works with your schedule and don't forget that you are also going to be adjusting your food and becoming more conscious of your eating this week so try not to overwhelm yourself. The goal of week 1 is to successfully keep your exercise promises to yourself and be ready to increase this just a bit during week 2.

You might also like to be looking ahead at your goals for Month 2 and a great goal would be to regularly add in one of your other types of exercise...maybe the regular ab work for example.

Further looking ahead might include Month 3 adding regular strength training into your routine.

So, knowing this, your first 4 weeks or so would really be all about cardio. Work on increasing your distance and the amount of time that you are walking. (or whatever cardio you choose to do) Going into week 2 I would encourage you to be having five days with cardio and from there increasing your time so that by the time you hit month 2, you are comfortable with five 30-40 minutes (minimum) of cardio a week. This would be a great goal in my opinion and if you are also watching your calories, I'm very confident that you'd be going into Month 2 with a pretty significant weight loss.

If you have the ab goal to begin in Month 2, you may also want to start trying that out by the end of your Month 1...just so you can start to get a feel for how that is going to be.

Of course, feel free to adapt any of this to suit your own abilities and motivation level. Certainly you can do more and the more you are able to do, the faster the weight will come off. I just want to stress that I want this to be changes for your life and not just a period of time while you are losing the weight.

Now we'll break down each of the three types of exercise and I will share with you what has worked for me.

Cardio

As mentioned in the section about finding something you love, this can be a critical piece to your success. Of course it is much easier to exercise long term when you actually enjoy what it is you are doing. If that is far off for you, the best advice that I can give you is to find something that is tolerable and can be relatively easy for you to complete on a regular basis. I predict once you start to see the benefits and the weight loss, you WILL begin to enjoy your workouts at least on some level.

There are so many things you can do to get your heart rate up and your body moving. The factors that may determine what you choose to do might have to do with cost and how accessible certain things are. For example, if cost isn't really an issue for you and you think you would be very motivated going to that cool new gym after work, by all means go for it. If cost is an issue and you're having a hard time imagining moving your body for long periods of time, start with walking in your neighborhood like I did. This is one of the easiest ways to get started and you can easily increase the level of difficulty with your own walking routine.

Decide if you'd prefer to workout inside, as the case of a local gym or outside in the fresh air. This may depend on what time of year it is and the climate conditions in your part of the country. If you love to bike or walk outside and you live somewhere where there will be a rough winter coming up, you'll probably want to come up with some good indoor alternatives for this time of year. Don't forget that you can also do a lot with great DVDs in your own living room. I personally recommend anything with Jillian Michaels does and I will include some links to my favorites in the resource section.

When I first started my weight loss plan, I chose to walk for my cardio exercise. This was cheap, easy and it got me outside. I also really enjoy listening to my iPod when I walk and started listening to a lot of great podcasts and things that motivated me which was a great second benefit to getting out for a walk.

Later, as I mentioned, I bought a bicycle and this became the main cardio exercise for me. I was able to increase my time significantly on the bike and would sometimes go for a 2-3 hour ride in the mornings which was a great way to start my day.

Over time walking, or the exercise you choose, will become much easier and you'll need to push yourself a bit more to get the same benefits of getting your heart rate up. You can do this by increasing your time or distance, your incline or by increasing your speed. All of these are very easy to do if you are working out on a treadmill. If you are walking outside, you may need to be a bit more intentional about creating some challenge with your walk. You could add dumb bells or ankle weights to your walking routine for example.

Probably the best thing you can do to keep your cardio routine interesting is to mix it up a bit from week to week. It is also practical to change up your routine to keep getting the benefits of losing weight because your body might need a little surprise now and then to get your metabolism going and continue losing weight.

My normal cardio goal is to do a minimum of 5 sessions of cardio a week for at least 40 minutes. When I was in intense weight loss mode, I would often do a lot more than this. I would maybe go for a long bike ride in the morning and then also get in a 30-40 minute walk in the evening. You design a routine that will work for you but of all the exercise you do, don't skimp on getting your cardio in if you really want to see some weight loss on the scale.

I will link to some calorie management tools in the resource section that you might want to check out. They track your calorie burn as well as the calories you consume on a regular basis.

Next we'll talk about the strength training portion of the exercise routine.

Strength Training

I can not stress the importance of doing strength training as part of your normal workout routine early on. I really believe that it was critical to my body getting in shape and it will allow you the benefits of feeling strong and more toned as you go.

There are many ways that you can incorporate strength training into your routine. If you already belong to a gym, this will be the logical place to start as most gyms have every piece of equipment you would need to develop a great routine for yourself. You may even want to consider hiring a personal trainer to get you started at the gym if that is something you can afford. It is critical that you are aware of your form when you are performing exercise with weights because you want the moves to be the most effective and you also do not want to risk injury, so even if you can't hire a trainer you should be able to talk to someone at the gym about correct use of the different types of machines.

I started out going to the small gym at my apartment complex to use the weights there. I then decided to create my own routine with dumb bells that I could do in my apartment. I like to do my weights while watching one of my favorite TV shows. The routine goes fast and it makes this goal something I can stick to each week.

You can also buy a very effective workout routine on a DVD and I will link to some in the resource section.

It's a good idea to give your body a day of rest when using weights. If you are working out both upper and lower body you could alternative these each day. I was mostly concerned about upper body strength so my normal strength training routine was Monday, Wednesday and Friday.

My typical upper body routine includes about 8 different exercises. It is difficult to explain each one here without images, but you can search online or start out with a good DVD if you're not sure about what to do. I do things like push-ups (easier style), chest presses and bicep curls just to give you an idea. If you start with one of Jillian Michael's DVDs (a word of warning - they are not easy!), you can always use them to learn the correct form and choose the best exercise to then design your own routine.

You should work up to doing 2-3 sets of these exercises and about 10-12 reps of each individual exercise. I find that 2 sets of dumb bells work well for me. I have a 5 lb set and a 10 lb set. You may want to start out lighter than 10 lbs at the beginning.

If you also want to include lower body strength training, you could do things such as lunges and squats for example. A good DVD will be able to give you ideas for both lower and upper body exercises.

I think it does take awhile to notice the benefits of working out with weights. You'll probably notice your weight loss before you notice an increase in muscle although do keep in mind that an increase in muscle can slow down your weight loss reflected on the scale in terms of numbers. Please do not let this discourage you because over time building your muscle is one of the best things you can do to make your body more efficient for losing the fat that is your real goal with all of this.

I think the most important thing is consistency here. Start as early as you can in your weight loss efforts, add it to your weekly goal list and just keep after it. You will be so thankful that you included strength training in your journey.

To help stay motivated, really notice the increase in your strength as you go. I found that I went from a single goal of wanting to not be fat to a goal of really wanting to feel fit and strong. I began to feel this way before I had really come close to my ultimate weight loss goal.

Next we'll go over how you can incorporate stretching and core work into your exercise routine.

Stretching and Core Work

I will admit to not really being the best example of stretching before and after my cardio workouts. It is a good idea to get in the habit of doing some typical stretching routines before and/or after you doing anything intense with your body. Here I am really referring to a more general type of stretching your body as part of your exercise routine.

I like to think of this portion of the three-pronged approach to getting my body in shape as the one that makes me longer. Of course you are not really adding inches (darn!) to your height but this can greatly improve your posture and certainly help you to feel more long and lean.

I love to do Pilates for this part of my routine, but you might also want to look at some type of yoga as many people love it and I believe it would offer many of the same benefits as I've gotten from Pilates.

I just started with, and still use, a very basic Pilates workout DVD. I will link to it in the resource section. My normal routine consisted of doing Pilates 2-3 times a week. The routine I do takes about 30-40 minutes and actually become one of the more relaxing parts of my week.

When I first started, I definitely could not get through all of the moves correctly and I dare say that I probably looked ridiculous! I certainly would never have done this in front of anyone back then at 250+ lbs or so. But over time, I could do all the exercises and I grew to love this part of my exercise routine for many reasons.

I found this a very peaceful thing to do. It can be a time to quiet your mind and just focus on your body. For that reason, I think the Pilates is another excellent way to get more in touch with your body if you've been in denial and not really experiencing your body as I had been. Over time notice how your body is changing as it becomes easier to do each of the exercises.

Next I want to move on to talk about ab work. Now I can imagine that if you have 100+ pounds to lose or if you are like many people who want to lose weight, a very noticeable place for losing that extra fat is going to be your stomach and waist.

Your ab work is going to be critical for developing a nice strong core. You will certainly get a lot of benefits in terms of working out your abs from the Pilates routine and also your strength training routine if you do the exercises correctly.

I had such an extreme inch loss in my stomach and waist that I thought it was worth mentioning this as a part of your normal routine.

I swear by a little workout called the '8 Min Abs". It is totally dated in terms of style - we're talking the 80's here. What I love about this routine is that it is ONLY 8 minutes long! I mean, who can't do an 8 minute routine on a regular basis, right? I just made the commitment to be consistent with this routine 5 days a week. For me this was Monday-Friday and I pretty much just said to myself that I would not have lunch before I did this routine. Knock it out day after day and experience real success with your abs.

A word of warning when you are just starting....that short little 8 minute workout is going to take forever AND you are going to feel it! Don't be discouraged and don't give up! Make this part of a process with a goal of doing the full 8 minutes without stopping. I also would encourage you to do some of each exercise rather than skipping whole portions. When you are just starting out, you also might not be able to do it 2 days in a row without rest because your abs will be sore. Do what you can but keep at it. I promise you that you will not regret it and you will be able to do this routine without problem in no time.

I also want to mention that there are other quick routines such as this available if you can't find this specific one. I will link to a few idea in the resource section for you.

Building up your core will contribute a lot to your success overall, so I encourage you to include this as part of your routine for losing weight and getting fit.

Next, we'll cover a section about creating some peace within your normal routine..hey, I know you could use some!

Create Peace in Your Routine

Though this section doesn't specifically speak to exercise and losing weight, I do want to mention a few ideas here because I think it can play a big role in developing a renewed sense of self esteem and reminding yourself of who you are meant to be in this world.

My approach to this comes from that of a Christian, but if that is not your belief system you can certainly incorporate mediation or stillness into your life in whatever way works for you. If this section of the book is not your cup of tea, feel free to move on..it's short.

I really believe in starting my day with prayer and reading my bible. I'm not saying I do this every day and I'm certainly not legalistic in any way when it comes to my Christianity and personal relationship with God.

I've already shared in a previous book that one of my biggest issues with my weight is that I felt like I was not being the person that God intended me to be. I'd allowed my weight to effect so much of my life and I knew it held me back from pursuing bigger dreams and goals for my life.

Starting my day with prayer and the bible centers me with my goals and what I believe are God's purposes for me. It is also a time of gratitude and seeking God for His strength to help me continue my efforts.

Regardless of what you might think, I definitely believe that there is a particular purpose to YOUR life. THAT'S really want I want for you…to be more of who you were meant to be. I'm guessing that your weight might also be hindering this for you, as it was for me.

Prayer, reading the bible or other spiritual books and meditation of some sort will help to quiet your mind and remind yourself of why you are putting in the effort each day to change your life. Consider incorporating some type of quiet time into your own morning routine as a way of centering yourself before you begin your day.

More peace in our lives is a good thing!

Next, we'll go over some ideas for finding the inspiration to keep you going

Finding Inspiration

The second book of the series on motivation was one of my favorites to write. I really encourage you to pick that one up if you feel like lacking the motivation to get started is your biggest issue.

Here I do want to go over some ideas specific to finding inspiration when it comes to losing weight and sticking with your exercise program as a key component to that process.

Create something visual.

Find pictures of bodies that you love. This is not to encourage you to want to be just like anyone else or have some kind of unrealistic expectation. Personally I find strong female bodies that are fit and lean very inspiring. You can either create a physical collage or vision board with images or use Pinterest as a way to create an online vision board for yourself.

Discover what will inspire you to keep going on the days when you really don't feel like it.

This really goes back to discovering what your bigger goals and vision for your life might be. This might be some of those things that you feel are being held back because of your weight. For me, for example, I have a big dream to be location independent starting with a move to Thailand and I definitely feel that my weight has been one factor that has kept me from doing that before now. I know that this is mostly in my head, but a factor nonetheless and one way that being overweight has affected me.

Keep your goals in front of you.

Having clear written goals that you can easily put in front of you can help to encourage and inspire you on those days when you just don't feel like going to the gym or heading out for your walk. Sometimes it is really just a simple matter of doing it so that you can cross if off your weekly goal or to-do list.

Exercise with a another person or a group.

Sometimes enlisting the support of a friend to workout with can be a big source of motivation for getting you to your workouts. Many times we will keep our commitments to another person before we would keep a commitment to ourselves to workout. I do encourage you to change this though. Meaning, make your commitments to yourself THE most important thing throughout this process. You also might be able to find a local group to workout with on a regular basis which can be fun. Consider looking online for a Meet-up group for example or on Craigslist (always be smart and keep safety in mind). There may be a group interested in weekly walks or hikes as an example and this can also be a social time to look forward to during your week.

Build a support network for inspiration.

Another great source of inspiration can come from meeting other people online who are also focused on weight loss goals. With all of the different social media sites out there such as Twitter, Facebook and weight loss specific blogs and forums it can be very easy to connect with other people. This can be a great source of motivation on those days when you don't feel like sticking to your exercise goals.

Really focus on putting a plan together that will keep you focused and in forward motion when it comes to exercise and achieving your own weight loss goals.

Listen, I don't want you to think that I am perfect with all of this. I'm not and definitely have my days when I give in to the thought of not keeping to my exercise commitment for a given day. As is with the eating goals, the MOST important thing will be what you do NEXT after a day like this. Do NOT let it derail all of your efforts. If you can get back on track quickly after skipping one of your intended goals, you will be fine. I promise you this.

Next, will talk about the fun part of recognizing all of your successes!

Pay Attention to Your Success

I think that for many of us, when we have a lot of weight to lose, it can be difficult to stop beating ourself up and looking at the long journey ahead.

I really encourage you to FIND things to feel good about. This really is a process and you're going to be taking some big steps to creating real change in your life. It's not always going to be easy but it will be worth it. I promise you that.

Find ways to celebrate your milestones as you go along your own journey. I'm not just talking about pounds lost here. I'm also talking about ways that you can mark the milestones of your exercise journey. You decide what those will be, but as an example you know that ab routine we talked about earlier? Celebrate the day you get through the WHOLE 8 minutes of it without stopping. You will deserve it!

I also want to encourage you to REALLY pay attention to how you are feeling once you start exercising and eating healthy foods.

I say this because there will be days you might be frustrated at how slow the weight is coming off or how long it is taking. During these times, if you focus on how much better you are feeling (you will be feeling better) then this is cause for recognition and celebration for how far you've come and your commitment to achieving your ultimate weight loss and fitness goals.

You will get there! It's exciting and the journey should be enjoyed as well as your end results!

Resources and Apps

There are many apps available for use on your smartphone or computer than can make the process of tracking your exercise and calorie burn easy and fun. Here are some that I would suggest you look at if you have an interest in this.

Calorie Management Systems:

bodybugg® Calorie Management System

This is a system that helps you to track the amount of calories that you consume as well as burn. It include an armband and a subscription based application service that is accessible via smartphone application or online. You also have the option to see your progress within the included display unit.

24hourfitness.com/training/bodybugg/

The Biggest Loser® SLIMCOACH™ and Polar WearLink® + transmitter

These two items also help you to track your calories, both consumed and burned. Visually, it is very easy to see when you hit your targets because the goal is to turn the Health Circle found on the device from red to green.

nbcuniversalstore.com

NIKE Fuelband

This is a similar tool in the form of a simple band that you wear around your wrist. This device tracks your movement and your progress towards a daily goal that you set. Once you've achieved your set movement goal for the day, the image on the device or software will turn green. You can either track your progress on your computer or with the smartphone app.

nike.com/fuelband/

Various Exercise DVDs:

Jillian Michaels

I would recommend anything with Jillian Michaels if you want to get a very effective workout in. It won't be easy to get through them at first, but stick with it and you're sure to notice results.

Jillian Michaels: Banish Fat, Boost Metabolism

Jillian Michaels: No More Trouble Zones

Jillian Michaels - 30 Day Shred

Jillian Michaels: Shred-It With Weights

Jillian Michaels: Yoga Meltdown

Ana Caban

There are a lot of various Pilates DVDs (Yoga) that you can check out. I personally like the style of Ana Caban so I will list a few of hers here.

Pilates - Beginning Mat Workout

Pilates Intermediate Mat Workout

Pilates Core Challenge with Ana Caban

8 Minute Abs

I can only find the VHS version of this on Amazon right now, but I will link to it in case you can find it somewhere else. There are a few other sets that include exercises for other parts of the body which I will also link to below.

8 Minute Abs [VHS]

8 Minute Workouts: Arms/Abs/Buns/Legs

:08 Min Core Workouts: Abs, Arms, Thighs, Buns and Stretch

Book 6: Getting Back on Track After Gaining Weight

A Note from Paula...

My working title for this book in the series has been the "Oops Edition".

How does one go from losing over 100 lbs (120 lbs to be exact!) to gaining almost half of the weight back AND still feel ready to put the gloves back on?

One of my biggest goals in writing this series is to help others who might be in a similar position as me with their weight, motivation and self esteem. One of my biggest intentions in doing this is to be as transparent and real with you as I can be.

I don't want to be that person who is selling you a formula for losing weight fast and fixing your life, yet hiding behind my own weight and insecurities. I will tell you straight out that you and I are very much the same. I'm not perfect in this and I like to call myself a work-in-progress for sure.

So my story continues as someone who DID lose 120 lbs by age 40, as was my original goal. At age 42 (my how time flies!), I found myself looking at a weight gain of almost half that weight. WOW! How could this have happened and what would I do about it?

Depending on when you are reading this, you might be joining me in this part of my journey to lose those 50 lbs and we really can do this together. (Be sure to send me a note - best place to connect would be via the Facebook page or my website - link at the end of the book)

The good news is that if I (or you) managed to lose 120 lbs of weight in a way that was healthy and for the most part not too difficult, we can do it again and do it for good.

The plan as laid out in the previous books of the series is solid. I know that for sure. It is doable, healthy and actually pretty fun. So the solution is about moving forward in that plan as opposed to trying to find another fad diet or quick weight loss gimmick that will probably work in the short term only, but we want lasting results here.

The real question isn't so much about losing the weight as it is in recognizing (without OVER analyzing) what went wrong and how to NOT do this in the future.

I want lasting change for me and I want lasting change for you. This means being able to cope with whatever life throws us without turning to food and by continuing to always aim for health.

This book is meant to help you to find the motivation to get back to your weight loss plan and to learn from past mistakes so that your weight gain is merely just another stepping stone to your ultimate goal, rather than an excuse to completely give up on changing your life.

If I can do this, so can you. Let's do it together.

In Book 6, I'd like to share with you what has worked for me in terms of getting back on track after a significant weight gain. You have the choice right now to continue down a path of destruction and depression or of getting back on track to being healthy and continuing to change your life.

This section is meant to be a blueprint to help with the motivation you need to get back on track after a weight gain.

To YOUR success,

Paula

What Happened?

How did it happen? How is it that one can go through all of the effort to lose over 100 lbs, only to be staring in the mirror at a 50 lb weight gain 2 years later.

Yes, this is my real story. I'm not proud of the fact that I had gained back that amount of weight. If I really think about it, it drives me pretty crazy because nothing felt as good to me as being in a body that was healthy and fit.

So what did happen in my case? Life happened for sure…it has or will for you too.

I lost a job, went through a few moves, had a few relationship issues…I could probably think of a few more reasons (excuses?), but you get the picture.

I am not one to dwell on things that are negative. I'm really more of a "glass is half full", "pick myself up by the bootstraps" kinda gal but I tell you these things so you get an idea of where life had taken me after the big weight loss.

I was less equipped to deal with this than I had thought. I obviously had the tools but I didn't really have a good action plan in place for dealing with the rough patches of life.

I allowed myself to slip back into some unhealthy eating habits and along with it an attitude of not caring as much. This was a textbook formula for weight gain.

I've learned some BIG lessons in this process. I am still learning as I go and as I change my life for the better.

I want you to pick yourself up also and vow to make this a part of the learning process. A weight gain, even after such a big loss, doesn't need to define you or your level of success with your own challenge to get healthy. USE this as just another stepping stone. IF you learn from it, you can move forward in a way that is healthy and a way that will bring you closer to long term success with your own weight loss.

If you find yourself in a similar position as me, I'm pretty sure that you've been knocking yourself around a bit when it comes to self talk and how you are feeling about yourself right now.

In the next section, I'm going to work to convince you to stop that nonsense. It's not useful and we need some new tools…new, positive self talk to get us back on track.

Not Beating Yourself Up

This is really a crucial part of the process. Can you vow to stop beating yourself up about your weight gain and the mistakes you've made? Can you make this promise today?

It really is not useful for you and I want you to start filling your mind…your entire being with every thought that is positive from this point on.

Yes, we are going to look at the mistakes we've made and how they did lead up to a weight gain BUT we are not doing this to punish ourselves. The motivation needs to come from a place of usefulness in terms of our continued journey on a path to being healthy and fit.

We can't be in denial about what got us here, so we do need to face it head on, but it is always about knowledge and change. Can you love yourself enough to be critical when it comes to analyzing the mistakes WITHOUT being critical of yourself. I know this can be difficult, but you don't have to beat yourself up about anything. Just refuse to do it any more.

This is all a process…a journey that we're on. We really have the opportunity to choose to look at the weight gain and mistakes as a way to learn and not throw our hands up in defeat. Just because you may have lost and then gained back weight in the past, it doesn't mean that this has to be the future for you. Only you get to decide that and you can choose optimism and knowledge and being about the business of learning from your mistakes as a way to keep moving forward towards your ultimate weight loss and health goals.

Now that we are DONE with any negativity and beating ourselves up (You're done with that, right?), let's take a look at what actually happened.

We'll start with what we've been doing right of course. ;)

Look at the Positives

Before we look at the mistakes we made and what led to our weight gain, I want you to dig deep and think about the things you've been doing right these past months.

If you've managed to lose a significant amount of weight prior to your recent weight gain, I would almost bet money on the fact that you did manage to keep doing a few things right. Please tell me it's so. (I'm winking as I type this, because I KNOW how easy it can be to "slip" into old patterns of living and "forget" the person we've become.)

I did manage to do a few things right. Thank goodness, or I'm pretty sure I would be looking at an even bigger weight gain.

Miracles of all miracles, throughout my weight loss I actually DID create an awesome habit of exercising regularly! Did you do this too?

I've managed to continue to do my cardio, strength training and ab work on a very consistent basis. Sure, there were day (sometimes weeks) that I missed, but overall this is something that has continued to be a regular part of my life. I consider this a huge success, so well done there.

Had I not been exercising, I'm very sure I would have gained back the 50 lbs sooner than what I did.

I continued to drink adequate amounts of water and eat much of the same healthy foods that I had been eating during my weight loss. (Mind you, there were "unhealthy" foods also, but we'll deal with that in the next section.)

I was in much "less" denial about my weight than I had been in past years. (Oh there was a bit of denial as the numbers increased on the scale for sure, but I've been worse in this regard.)

I didn't allow myself to buy new clothes in bigger sizes except for what was absolutely necessary. This could be easier for me than some people as I work from home and my wardrobe is not really a big part of my life. This is also a negative aspect which I will cover in the next section.

Now it's your turn…try as hard as you can to not be in "beat myself up mode" and think about what things you HAVE been doing well. In what ways have you not completely gone back to square one with this process?

If by chance, you really can't find one good thing you've been doing…I forgive you. Please forgive yourself.

It doesn't mean success is not meant for you or that you won't reach your own goal of becoming healthy and fit. It just means you're getting ready to be "real" with yourself and make a promise to be MORE mindful and MORE present in your body from now on. That, I know you can do.

Now we're ready to deal with our mistakes…deep breath, it's OK.

What Were the Mistakes?

OK, this section might call for a deep breathe. We can do it. We're going to get through it together.

Where did we go wrong?

Was it that first trip to the local fast food place? Was it that week off on vacation? When I made the move (again) cross country, I didn't really have a good plan in place. Is that when it happened? Then I had a relationship go sour that definitely did my head in for a bit. Was it then that I threw in the towel and decided I didn't care about my health any more? I lost a job and felt like a complete loser for a time as I dealt with some financial issues. THAT definitely was a depressing time and I can see where that may have been a big turning point for me.

I'm being a bit silly in sharing all of that. (Well, silly isn't really a good word as all of those things DID happen and it was anything but silly at the time.)

My point is that life happened to me. Of course there were a lot of good things that happened during that same time period, but the point is that life can be a bit of a roller coaster. We know that. Losing weight and getting healthy does NOT make our lives perfect. We will still need to learn how to deal with life's challenges.

The thing to be acutely aware of if you have a challenge with overeating and your weight, is that we tend to deal with life's issues by finding comfort in food and old habits that ultimately led to us being very fat. It is critical that we learn new behaviors for dealing with these aspects of life because food is only a short term fix that can lead to a longer term problem if we let it get out of hand.

So, it's time to really think about where our mistakes were during this time. This is NOT about beating ourselves up. This is about using the data for information to create a plan for the future. We need a plan at least for a period of time. This will be something we can turn to when we are faced with the bumps in the road of life and something that will help us to NOT get so far off track that it is a struggle to get back to all of our healthy and new ways of being.

Here are some of my mistakes.

When I started gaining weight, I stopped tracking my calories.

I let an infrequent visit to a fast food place lead to more of a regular habit.

I gave myself permission to overindulge when I was PMS or generally feeling down.

I became less organized with my weekly meal planning and grocery shopping.

I stopped weighing myself regularly.

I stopped wearing my jeans. (Spent most of my time in sweats or PJs)

I stopped writing my blog on a regular basis. (Apparently blogging had really helped me to be accountable!)

So there are some of my biggies. Do you have your list?

It is important that we do this step to be able to learn and grow from it as we move on. It's really the only way to go forward in a way that will lead to success. I want to stress that I am NOT into OVER analyzing this. I just think we need to acknowledge the past mistakes so that we can be ACTIVE in making a plan for the future that includes a blueprint for how we will tackle each of these things WHEN they do come up again. They WILL come up again!

I also want to take a moment to say that although I am not qualified at all to analyze the bigger issues of why you might be falling back into unhealthy patterns, I am a huge advocate in seeking therapy to help recognize what some of these deeper issues might be. There is definitely a time and a place for a good therapist and personally I believe that everyone can benefit from this at some point in their life. I had a therapist for several years and the experience completely changed my life.

Also, it is worth saying that there might be very valid reason why food and weight gain has become a coping mechanism for someone. Only you know the issues of your past and I just want to give you the permission and support to seek out help for things that are truly beyond your ability to help yourself. That would be the most loving thing you could do for yourself.

In the next section, we'll talk about how we are going to muster up the motivation to get back on track again! We ARE doing this!

How to Get Back to It

In terms of our actual steps, I'm not suggesting anything different here than what I've been outlining in the previous books.

This is NOT the time to turn to a fast diet, a liquid diet or anything other than what is healthy and what you know has worked for you in the past in terms of losing the weight.

In terms of this series, it means:

1. Creating a revised strategy (Book 1: Creating YOUR Plan for Weight Loss Success)

2. Revisiting the images, vision board, videos and other things we created to motivate ourselves in the beginning (Book 2: How to Find the Motivation to Lose Weight and Get Healthy)

3. Designing some new goals and a plan of action (Book 3: Goal Setting for Weight Loss)

4. Creating a menu and grocery list for the upcoming week and a new commitment to recording calories (Book 4: Eating for Weight Loss)

5. Creating exercise goals for the upcoming week and putting them on the calendar (Book 5: Exercise for Weight Loss)

Now, what you might need from me here is a good dose of motivation…all the reasons why I know you CAN do this.

Actually if you've lost any amount of weight close to what I had lost, the good news is that you were just there, right? I'm betting that if you close your eyes and think back to your lowest weight on the journey, you can remember how you were feeling.

THIS needs to be your motivation during the trying times of getting back to all of your healthy habits during Week 1. Remember when you were starting out? It's really that critical Week 1 that is the tipping point. If you can manage to just hang on, put your head down and stick to your goals for that first full week, chances are you'll be sailing towards continued weight loss after that point.

So pretty much the pep talk is summed up as "just do it". Get through Week 1 and you're moving back along your right path.

OK, I know it may not be as easy as all that, but you get what I mean. You really can turn this around and if we decide to learn from our past mistakes, there isn't a reason why the scale ever needs to go back in that "other" direction again. (at least not by much, right?)

In the next section, I'll go over some strategies for creating a plan that will deal with future challenges and how we can insure that we will never get this off track again.

A New Plan for Lasting Success

Here is where we want to revisit each of our "mistakes" and create a plan for strategies for dealing with these things in the future. They WILL come up again…you can bet on that. The key to success will be staying conscious about the choices we make and not being in denial about the repercussions (potential weight gain) of choosing the unhealthy choice.

I will start by using my mis-steps as an example. I'm guessing these may actually be similar to yours. See how much alike we are? ;)

When I started gaining weight, I stopped tracking my calories.

1. Track calories on a daily/weekly basis. Re-commit to tracking my calories on a daily/weekly basis. I use the iPhone app Lose It which makes it really easy. The real challenge with this for me is not throwing in the towel on the calorie counting as soon as I go over the calories on a given day. Really the commitment should be to track the calories REGARDLESS of how the day is going. THIS is what keeps one/me out of denial!

If I do need a break (sometimes this can get old for whatever reason), allow myself 2 days out of the month if/as needed without calorie counting. This should not be used as an excuse to go crazy with the food, but as a measure to see how we might get on without tracking down the road. I don't know about you, but I would love to foresee a future when I wouldn't have to track calories and eating the right amounts of foods would just be a completely natural thing for me.

I let an infrequent visit to a fast food place lead to more of a regular habit.

2. Know and limit the things that are your "triggers" for old habits. This is an area I really need to stay on top of because for me it can be a slippery slope. I think we all have different "triggers" when it comes to foods or habits that can lead to a downward spiral if we are not fully conscious. I don't want to veto any food completely. For me, this just doesn't work long term. I would say that it's probably wise though to have at least a period of abstinence for fast food while I get back on track and start feeling stronger about my choices.

The next course of action for something like this might be to put a limit on it as a way of dealing with a potential issue longer term. I can imagine saying that I wouldn't have fast food more than 2 times a month for example. Another way to deal with this would be to have a plan for exactly what one's menu choices would be during a fast food or other restaurant visit. I tend to not go so much because of convenience as I do to give in to craving a particular item on the menu, but for someone who eats out more regularly because of necessity, advance planning and healthy food selection is definitely the way to curb this trigger point.

I gave myself permission to overindulge when I was PMS or generally feeling down.

3. Have a plan in place for things you can do to feel better when you are dealing with PMS or a general feeling of uneasiness. So the reality (if you're a woman) is that PMS is probably not going away any time soon. I can pretty much count on this every month. Grrr.. What I do know though is that when I am exercising regularly and eating healthy, the symptoms are definitely lessoned and many of my cravings and crazy moments can be somewhat tamed. This means that a resolution for this challenge might be just in the re-commitment to focusing on the weight loss strategy again. I can also do a better job of tracking and planning for this time by having options on hand that are a treat (like my favorite low fat ice cream or 100 calorie snacks), but won't break the calorie budget for the week.

In term of emotionally low times, I know that there are certain healthy things that I can do that will help to bring me out of a down mood. Exercise is an excellent plan for an occasion such as that. It's hard to remain depressed while out on your bike in the sunshine for a nice 2 hour ride. Sometimes during a down time, I will also just let myself be somewhat "lazier" than normal BUT only for the day. It could be a good occasion for a nice movie marathon for example. This is fine as long as a bunch of junk food (or alcohol!) doesn't also make its way into the mix.

I became less organized with my weekly meal planning and grocery shopping.

4. Be organized with your daily/weekly menu planning and grocery list. This means going back to basics and the commitment to planning out my healthy meals on a daily (if not weekly basis) and making sure that I am prepared with a list when I go grocery shopping. Along with this, don't shop while hungry and avoid impulse purchases which are less likely if we stick to the list. If you are feeling bored with all the foods you were eating previously, it might also be a great idea to explore some new recipes as a way to get back into your routine. Perhaps try a new favorite ethnic food that you love. There may even be a grocery store that caters more to different types of foods depending on how big of area you live in.

I stopped weighing myself regularly.

5. Weigh yourself once a week to stay on top of any weight gain. In my opinion, when it comes to mistakes and setting oneself up for denial, this is the biggest factor. If we avoid the scale, it's so much easier to just keep going along with our old habits. There is something about facing the reality of the number on the scale that can really stop us in our tracks which is what we want, right? Of course it is so much easier to deal with any weight gain when you catch it very early. My strategy is to weigh myself a minimum of once a week no matter what.

I stopped wearing my jeans. (Spent most of my time in sweats or PJs)

6. Do not only wear clothes that are more "forgiving" of weight gain - sweats and PJs as an example. For me, this was a very easy mistake to make because I work from home and spend a lot of time alone. This translates into being completely comfortable and rarely getting dressed up or putting on make-up. In theory, I have no issue with this and love the freedom and the fact that I can spend time doing other things beside worrying too much about my day-to-day appearance. The obvious downside to this is it's very easy to not really notice putting on 5 lbs or so if you are constantly in pants that have elastic or a drawstring. Doh! The solution is to put the jeans on (Heck, maybe even some make-up) a few times a week at least for a period of time. Wearing your jeans every once in awhile is a sure way to keep those added inches in check.

I stopped writing my blog on a regular basis. (Apparently blogging had really helped me to be accountable!)

7. Have some form of accountability to help with support. You may or may not be blogging about your personal life or weight loss struggle. Hopefully if you are not, you do have at least one person in your life who is able to be an accountability partner for you. Being accountable to another person (or the blogosphere!) can be a really big help when it comes to staying on track with your weight loss efforts. It can be critical to create some kind of support system for yourself as you begin your journey and equally as critical to be able to reach out to others when you do need some added motivation and support. Commit to sharing your struggle with someone else who will understand what you are going through. If you want to take it a step further, you can set up your own online presence in the form of a personal blog or even through a Facebook page which is free and doesn't require a lot of technical experience.

Additional Suggestions for Staying on Track Long Term:

8. Know your weight gain limit. This is really more about when we get into the maintenance phase after reaching our ultimate weight loss goal, but I did want to mention this as a critical point for not gaining the weight back. Of course we would all love to not have to worry about gaining weight or fluctuations with the numbers we see on the scale, but that is just not realistic. Especially for women, our weight can definitely fluctuate with PMS and bloating. I suggest that as you continue to weigh yourself at least once a week, have a weight range rather than one particular number that you are attached to. Having said this, you should also have an upper number in mind that will trigger some different patterns. If you nip this right away, a 5 lb gain does not have to turn into 10 lbs and you can very easily get that off again by watching your calories and exercise for the next few weeks.

9. Take the time to create a vision board for your future and keep it in front of you for inspiration. Having something visual for motivation can really help you to keep on track with your commitment and goals. When you feel yourself slipping, take the time to really look at that visual representation that you've created for the life you want to have. You can change your life. Do what you need to do to keep that fire burning.

10. Design a special reward that will help you get back on track with your weight loss efforts. As an example, maybe you could schedule a nice little trip 3 months from now. Las Vegas or a spa weekend comes to mind depending on what types of activities you are into. If travel doesn't really suit you, another idea might be to save up for a really cute new outfit for a special event you have coming up or for no other reason than having a nice little addition for your current wardrobe. Choose a reward that has meaning for you and one that will inspire you to keep going with your efforts.

If no one else understands or believes that you can do this, I want you to know that I am your cheerleader! ;) Read on my friend...

I Believe in You

I know what it's like to feel like you're all alone in your weight loss struggle. You look around you at all of the people in your life who seem to have it so together and at times you feel like you are standing alone.

I've been there even though I KNOW I have friends and family who love and support me.

I think only someone who has been through this journey and lived as an obese person can truly understand all of the pain and struggle one goes through during this process. This is not to say other people don't also have their issues. They do for sure. I know plenty of people who are thin and unhappy so being thin or fit is not the answer to finding happiness.

When we are obese, we wear our "issue" for everyone to see…to judge. It's a fact. It's there.

I just want to take this opportunity to tell you that I do believe that you can do this…the same way that I believe this for myself.

We have the desire and the knowledge to make a significant change in our lives. If you are coming from a recent gain after a big loss, you already know what it feels like to experience some success with feeling fit and lighter. Dig deep and remember how that felt. How badly do you want that again?

I want that for you…I'm believing that for you and I hope you are also ready to make the commitment.

Let's do this!

Next Steps

I hope that you have enjoyed reading the compilation guide of the series, "How to Lose 100 Pounds" and I also sincerely hope that it will inspire you to make healthy lasting changes for your own life.

I very much appreciate your reviews and comments as I love to put a name to those who are creating a healthy and happy life.

We're in this together and I want you to know that you have a cheerleader in me!

Good luck on your weight loss! I know that you can do this!

I'd love to hear from you.

Visit the site below to download my **FREE gift** to you - "Your Success Plan for Weight Loss." (And to be notified of new titles and special offers)

CelebrateWeightLoss.com

Please also join us on **FaceBook** - there is a great, supportive group of people there:

Facebook.com/howtolose100pounds

Twitter

Twitter.com/pseymour

To YOUR success,

Paula

Now Available in Audio

"How to Lose 100 Pounds" is now available as an audiobook!

You can listen to a free sample here:
Amazon.com/dp/B00II6504Y/

Visit the author website for additional audiobooks:

CelebrateWeightLoss.com

Additional Titles by P. Seymour

Visit CelebrateWeightLoss.com

****

Series "The Personal Transformation Project - Part 1: How to Feel Awesome!"

How to Be Happier: A Blueprint for Creating More Joy in Your Life

How to Be Motivated: A Blueprint for Increasing Your Motivation

How to Be Healthier: A Blueprint for Creating a Healthy Lifestyle

How to Be Confident: A Blueprint for Increasing Your Self-Confidence

How to Be Positive: A Blueprint for Developing a Positive Attitude

How to Be Relaxed: A Blueprint for Reducing Stress in Your Life

SAVE OVER 45% with the Compilation Guide!
(Includes ALL 6 Books Above)
The Personal Transformation Project: Part 1 How to Feel Awesome!
*Also available in paperback

Resolutions in the New Year...or Any Time: How to Make a Plan for Transformation

Legal Notices and Disclaimers:

NOT MEDICAL ADVICE

No part of this book is considered to be medical advice. You are strongly encouraged to seek the advice of a qualified, licensed and competent medical doctor before starting any exercise routine or changes to your diet.

ALL RIGHTS RESERVED

No part of this book may be altered in any form whatsoever, electronic or otherwise, including photocopying, recording, or by any informational storage or retrieval system without express written, dated and signed permission from the author.

DISCLAIMER AND/OR LEGAL NOTICES

The information presented here represents the view of the author as of the date of publication. Because of the rate with which conditions change, the author reserves the right to alter and update her opinion based on new conditions as applicable. This book is for informational purposes only. While every attempt has been made to verify the information provided in this book, neither the author nor her affiliates/partners assume any responsibility for errors, inaccuracies or omissions. Any slights of people or organizations are unintentional. You should be aware of any laws which govern business transactions or other business practices in your country and state. Any reference to any person or business whether living or dead is purely coincidental.

The purchaser or reader of this publication assumes responsibility for the use of these materials and information. Adherence to all applicable laws and regulations, federal, state, and local, governing professional licensing, business practices, advertising, and all other aspects of doing business in the United States or any other jurisdiction is the sole responsibility of the purchaser or reader.

The author and publisher assume no responsibility or liability whatsoever on the behalf of any purchaser or reader of these materials.